Compartment Syndrome

Cyril Mauffrey • David J. Hak
Murphy P. Martin III

Editors

Compartment Syndrome

A Guide to Diagnosis and Management

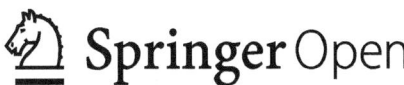

Editors
Cyril Mauffrey 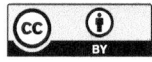, MD, FACS, FRCS
Professor of Orthopedic Surgery
Interim Director of Service
Department of Orthopedics
Denver Health Medical Center
Denver, CO
USA

David J. Hak, MD, MBA, FACS
Central Florida Regional Hospital
Hughston Orthopedic Trauma Group
Sanford, FL
USA

Murphy P. Martin III, MD
Assistant Professor
Department of Orthopedic Surgery
Tulane University School of Medicine
New Orleans, LA
USA

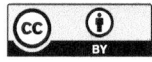

Preface

Despite the relatively high incidence of compartment syndrome and the fairly dismal outcomes, this condition remains poorly studied and understood. While the pathophysiology seems to be clear, an absolute diagnosis is at times virtually impossible. The conundrum of the timing of onset of symptoms and of the relationship between level of pain, symptoms, signs, and microscopic changes within the compartment remains a mystery. The aim of our open-access text was to review this condition to answer simple questions pertinent to compartment syndrome. We have gathered a group of experts in the field to provide an easily downloadable and accessible series of chapters. The book covers topics ranging from diagnosis to treatment and outcomes. We use the same format in each chapter to enhance the readers' experience. We hope that you will enjoy and learn. The open-access format will make this work available to low- and middle-income countries where surgeons do not always have the resources to fund such material.

We dedicate this work to our hardworking residents and fellows, without whom, our daily activities would not be as stimulating as they are.

Denver, CO, USA   Cyril Mauffrey
Sanford, FL, USA   David J. Hak
New Orleans, LA, USA   Murphy P. Martin III

Acknowledgments

We want to acknowledge our funding body AO North America for making this project possible.

Contents

Contributors

Amiethab Aiyer, MD University of Miami Hospital, Department of Orthopedic Surgery, Miami, FL, USA

Derek Ball, BSc (Hons), PhD School of Medicine, University of Aberdeen, Medical Sciences and Nutrition, Aberdeen, Aberdeenshire, UK

Jennifer L. Bruggers, MD Resurgens Orthopedics, Atlanta, GA, USA

Salih Colakoglu, MD Plastic Surgery Department, University of Colorado, Aurora, CO, USA

Charles M. Court-Brown, MD, FRCS (Ed), Orth University of Edinburgh, Edinburgh, UK

Andrew D. Duckworth, Bsc, FRCS Edinburgh Orthopedic Trauma Unit, Royal Infirmary of Edinburgh, Edinburgh, UK

Joshua L. Gary, MD University of Texas Health Science Center at Houston, McGovern Medical School, Department of Orthopedic Surgery, Houston, TX, USA

Peter V. Giannoudis, BSc, MB, MD, FRCS, FACS Academic Department of Trauma and Orthopedics, School of Medicine, University of Leeds, NIHR Leeds Biomedical Research Center, Chapel Allerton Hospital, Leeds Teaching Hospitals NHS Trust, Leeds, UK

David J. Hak, MD, MBA Hughston Orthopedic Trauma Group, Central Florida Regional Hospital, Sanford, FL, USA

Sascha Halvachizadeh, MD University Hospital Zurich, Trauma Department, Zurich, Zurich, Switzerland

Edward J. Harvey, MD, MSc, FRCSC McGill University, Michal and Renata Hornstein Chair in Surgical Excellence, Montreal General Hospital, Montreal, QC, Canada

Vasilios G. Igoumenou, MD First Department of Orthopedics, National and Kapodistrian University of Athens, School of Medicine, Athens, Attica, Greece

Kyros Ipaktchi, MD, FACS Orthopedic Department, Denver Health Medical Center, Denver, CO, USA

Kai Oliver Jensen, MD University Hospital Zurich, Trauma Department, Zurich, Zurich, Switzerland

Alan J. Johnstone, MB, ChB, FRCSE (Orth) Aberdeen Royal Infirmary & University of Aberdeen, Orthopedic Trauma Unit, Aberdeen, Grampian Region, UK

Anish R. Kadakia, MD University of Miami Hospital, Department of Orthopedic Surgery, Miami, FL, USA

Northwestern University, Northwestern Memorial Hospital, Chicago, IL, USA

Jonathan Kaplan, MD University of Miami Hospital, Department of Orthopedic Surgery, Miami, FL, USA

Orthopedic Specialty Institute, Orange, CA, USA

Zinon T. Kokkalis, MD Department of Orthopedics, University of Patras, Patras, Achaia, Greece

Christopher Lee, MD R Adams Cowley Shock Trauma Center, Department of Orthopedic Surgery, Baltimore, MA, USA

Virginia Commonwealth University, Department of Orthopedic Surgery, Trauma, Richmond, VA, USA

Carol A. Lin, MD, MA Cedars-Sinai Medical Center, Department of Orthopedic Surgery, Los Angeles, CA, USA

Milton T. M. Little, MD Cedars-Sinai Medical Center, Orthopedic Surgery Department, Cedars-Sinai Orthopedic Center, Los Angeles, CA, USA

Julian G. Lugo-Pico, MD University of Miami Hospital, Department of Orthopedic Surgery, Miami, FL, USA

University of Miami/Jackson Memorial Hospital, Miami, FL, USA

Douglas W. Lundy, MD, MBA, FACS Resurgens Orthopedics, Atlanta, GA, USA

Michael Maher, MD Denver Health Medical Center, Department of Orthopedic Trauma, Denver, CO, USA

Cyril Mauffrey, MD, FACS, FRCS Department of Orthopedic Surgery, Denver Health Medical Center, Denver, CO, USA

Andreas F. Mavrogenis, MD First Department of Orthopedics, National and Kapodistrian University of Athens, School of Medicine, Athens, Attica, Greece

Margaret M. McQueen, MD, FRCSEd(orth) University of Edinburgh, Edinburgh, UK

Geraldine Merle, PhD Montreal General Hospital, Montreal, QC, Canada

Sean Morell, MD Orthopedic Department, University of Colorado, Aurora, CO, USA

Robert V. O'Toole, MD, MS R Adams Cowley Shock Trauma Center, Department of Orthopedic Surgery, Baltimore, MA, USA

Ioannis V. Papachristos, MD, MSc Leeds Teaching Hospitals NHS Trust, Department of Trauma and Orthopedics, Leeds General Infirmary, Leeds, UK

Hans-Christoph Pape, MD, FACS University Hospital Zurich, Trauma Department, Zurich, Zurich, Switzerland

Joshua A. Parry, MD, MS Denver Health Medical Center, Department of Orthopedics, Denver, CO, USA

Andrew H. Schmidt, MD University of Minnesota, Minneapolis, MN, USA

Department of Orthopedic Surgery, Hennepin Healthcare, Minneapolis, MN, USA

Cody M. Tillinghast, MD University of Texas Health Science Center at Houston, McGovern Medical School, Department of Orthopedic Surgery, Houston, TX, USA

Mark S. Vrahas, MD, MHCDS Cedars-Sinai Medical Center, Department of Orthopedic Surgery, Los Angeles, CA, USA

Jessica Wingfield, MD Orthopedic Department, University of Colorado, Aurora, CO, USA

Chapter 1
Diagnostic Dilemma for the Orthopedic Surgeon

Michael Maher and Cyril Mauffrey

Background

1. Compartment syndrome is associated with serious long-term morbidity.
2. Appropriate treatment is invasive and involves its own risks.
3. The presentation of compartment syndrome is variable.
4. The diagnosis of compartment syndrome relies largely on clinical findings.
5. Pressure monitoring may provide supplemental but imperfect diagnostic guidance.

The diagnosis and management of compartment syndrome represents a dilemma for clinicians. A major cause of concern in treating compartment syndrome is the potentially devastating outcome if not treated effectively. Compartment syndrome results in ischemia within a fascial compartment that eventuates into necrosis of the tissues it encompasses. Sequelae of missed compartment syndrome include loss of function, contracture of joints, limb deformity, and painful neuropathies [1, 2]. These complications persist and significantly reduce quality of life. In light of this, the timely diagnosis and treatment of compartment syndrome is a focus of orthopedic surgery training. However, an inconsistency in practice remains. O'Toole et al. [3] demonstrated a wide variation between orthopedic surgeons, even within a single practice of orthopedic trauma specialists at a level I trauma center. A diagnostic rate of compartment syndrome for tibia fractures ranged from 2% to 24% depending on the surgeon who was on call. This demonstrates the lack of consensus and clarity with regard to diagnosis.

M. Maher
Denver Health Medical Center, Department of Orthopedic Trauma, Denver, CO, USA

C. Mauffrey (✉)
Department of Orthopedic Surgery, Denver Health Medical Center, Denver, CO, USA
e-mail: cyril.mauffrey@dhha.org

© The Author(s) 2019
C. Mauffrey et al. (eds.), *Compartment Syndrome*,
https://doi.org/10.1007/978-3-030-22331-1_1

1

The prognosis is grave in cases of missed compartment syndrome, but there are even severe repercussions for a diagnosis delayed by a matter of hours. If the treating surgeon correctly recognizes compartment syndrome, but attempts late release of the fascia over a necrotic compartment, the patient is subject to a high risk of infection and life-threatening complications [4]. Sheridan and Matsen report an infection rate of 46%, and an amputation rate of 21% after fasciotomy was delayed by 12 hours [5]. Only 2% of those patients treated on a delayed basis had a normal functioning extremity at final follow up, compared to 68% in those treated earlier. Reperfusion after severe muscle necrosis may further increase systemic effects. As myonecrosis develops and reperfusion is achieved, myoglobin is released into circulation, further contributing to myoglobinuria, metabolic acidosis, and hyperkalemia. This may lead to renal failure, shock, and cardiac events [6, 7]. Although fascial release is the appropriate treatment of acute compartment syndrome, clinicians must be aware of the dangers of late surgical intervention.

In addition to the serious consequences of missed or delayed treatment of acute compartment syndrome, clinicians and patients may face complications even in the setting of treatment with the correct technique and timing. A retrospective study looking at the long-term outcomes of fasciotomy placement by Fitzgerald et al. does not convey a completely benign procedure [8]. Reviewed outcomes of 164 patients over an 8-year period showed pain (10%), altered sensation (77%), dry skin (40%), pruritis (33%), discoloration (30%), swelling (13%), and muscle herniation (23%). Scarring of the extremities caused patients to keep extremity covered (23%), changed hobbies (28%), and even changed occupation (12%). Fasciotomy sites may also require the patient to undergo multiple interventions of attempted wound closure or grafting. In the setting of operative fractures, the placement of fasciotomy incisions may complicate surgical approach and increase risk of infection and nonunion of fracture sites.

In addition to the issues relating to the morbidity, complications, and time pressure of compartment syndrome, the diagnosis itself is rarely straightforward. Patients may present following a typical injury and exhibit classic symptoms, but they will likely include a constellation of positive and negative findings. The diagnostic dilemma of acute compartment syndrome is always present because it is a clinical diagnosis. The classic signs and symptoms of acute compartment syndrome are often listed as the 5 or 6 "Ps" including some variation of pain, pressure, pulselessness, paralysis, paresthesia, and pallor [1, 2, 5, 9]. Early descriptions of diagnosis of compartment syndrome begin with those of ischemic contracture in the upper extremity by Volkmann, followed by more recent observations in the lower extremity, such as those described by Seddon [1]. However, while describing the diagnostic "Ps" of compartment syndrome, Seddon noted that they were absent in over half of the cases he reviewed [10]. These diagnostic findings may simply be unavailable in a timely manner. Pain out of proportion or in response to passive stretch may be an early indicator for compartment syndrome, but is unreliable in cases where a patient is obtunded or experiencing a neural deficit. Other signs, such as pallor or paralysis, may be delayed to the point of being useless.

The pressure gradient within the fascial compartment exceeds perfusion pressure in order for compartment syndrome to set in. It is not often possible to specify when this threshold is reached, but we do know that the clinician only has a limited amount of time by that point. This threshold and the amount of time before irreversible damage is done has been a focus of study. A clear relationship between compartment pressure and blood pressure has been established with the use of animal models and observations of intra-compartmental pressures, tissue histology, oxygenation, and magnetic resonance spectroscopy [11, 12]. A study by Heckman et al. documented complete irreversible ischemic infarction of skeletal muscle by inducing elevated intra-compartmental pressures for 8 hours [8]. Variable recovery may be expected with earlier intervention. The threshold at which ischemia begins is difficult to predict. It may coincide with the traumatic event or set in insidiously. McQueen et al. [13] reported the average treatment of compartment syndrome 7 hours after manipulation and fixation in 13 cases with continuous monitoring and a delayed onset as late as 24 hours postoperatively. A late-onset variety of compartment syndrome has been reported as late as 4 days after an inciting event [6, 14].

Another factor adding to diagnostic difficulty of compartment syndrome is the myriad of injuries and conditions that may precede its onset. A classic scenario of acute compartment syndrome in the lower extremity is the result of a closed tibial shaft fracture [2, 15, 16]. However, compartment syndrome may develop with a huge variety of situations. Possible etiologies may include open and closed fractures, vascular injury, burns, intravenous access leakage, contusion, coagulopathies, constrictive dressing, patient positioning during surgery, drug overdose or animal bites [17]. Therefore, clinicians cannot rely on specific presentation factors to rule out developing compartment syndrome. The most common causes of acute compartment syndrome, as described in a series presented by McQueen et al. [18], was fracture (69%) followed by soft tissue injury without fracture (23.2%). The most common fractures observed were tibial diaphysis (36%) and distal radius (9.8%).

Compartment syndrome is a stressful situation for the patient and clinician. There exists a combination of significant morbidity, risks of invasive intervention, time limitations, and variations in presentation. Unfortunately, there is also the awareness that compartment syndrome and its sequelae are the source of a significant amount of litigation [19–21]. The prospect of undergoing a medical malpractice claim or suit is daunting and can be especially draining for physicians unaccustomed to the medicolegal process. It will likely create a significant cost in time, energy, finances, and emotional burden [22]. Orthopedic surgeons are a medical specialty at relatively higher risk of encountering medicolegal claims [23]. Given the high morbidity to patients, awards for plaintiffs or settlements may be large. One national database review of suits involving compartment syndrome found an average award for settlements out of court to be over 1 million dollars and average verdict awards for plaintiffs to be over 2 million dollars [17]. A review of claims involving compartment syndrome by Bhattacharyya and Vrahas found the average time commitment to resolve a claim to be 5.5 years [17].

Recommendations

The diagnosis of compartment syndrome is largely based on clinical judgment, history, and physical exam. Patient history in regard to mechanism of injury may be helpful in identifying factors that would increase risk of soft tissue injury such as crushing or high energy trauma. History may also include other medical risk factors such and coagulopathies or infusion injury. Findings on the exam typically focus on the presence of pain, pressure, pulselessness, paralysis, paresthesia, and pallor. These findings are especially instructive if they correspond to a specific compartment in question. The presence of firmness versus compressibility of a compartment is advantageous as it does not require consciousness or cooperation of a patient and may be the earliest manifestation of compartment syndrome. It is important to note that acute compartment syndrome is not a static process and cannot be adequately ruled out in a suspected case based on a single evaluation. Rather, it is advisable to include serial examinations, typically spaced 1–2 hours apart to ensure any changes may be detected and addressed in a timely manner [16].

Measurement of compartment pressures can be a useful tool in situations where the clinical picture is muddled. There are multiple techniques described for pressure monitoring, including slit catheter, wick catheter, infusion, and side port needle devices. Commercially available side-port needle devices have gained popularity with their ability to measure multiple compartments and ease of use [8, 14]. As the development of ischemia is dependent upon a differential between compartment pressure and perfusion pressure, the threshold at which compartment pressures should be considered dangerous is often described in comparison to diastolic pressures. This differential, commonly described as ΔP, was described in canine models with a critical pressure being within 20 mmHg of diastolic pressure, resulting permanent abnormalities noted in muscle tissue. In a prospective study, McQueen and Court-Brown observed 116 patients with tibial diaphyseal fractures who underwent continuous anterior compartment pressure monitoring for 24 hours [24]. They noted absolute pressures reaching as high as 50 mmHg in multiple patients, but only three met a fasciotomy threshold criteria of ΔP less than 30 mmHg. No other patients were noted to develop compartment syndrome, resulting in a ΔP less than 30 mmHg being widely accepted as a threshold for surgical intervention.

Limitations and Pitfalls

Although clinical findings are important in diagnosis of acute compartment syndrome, the predictive value of individual findings is low. One analysis of 4 prospective studies involving 132 cases of compartment syndrome found that the positive predictive value of individual findings such as pain, paresthesia, and paresis was low at 11–15%, but the likelihood of successful diagnosis did increase with multiple clinical findings. However, the negative predictive value was as high as 98% [25]. Therefore, the presence of individual clinical findings was not as useful as noting the absence of such findings, to rule out the presence of compartment syndrome.

The use of local nerve blocks, epidural or regional anesthesia, is not recommended in the setting of possible compartment syndrome. Local anesthetics may mask pain from increasing compartment pressures or neurologic symptoms that would usually alert clinicians [26]. Additionally, the use of epidural anesthesia may increase the risk of developing compartment syndrome as sympathetic blockade will increase local blood flow and possibly exacerbate intracompartmental pressure increases [27, 28].

In situations where clinical findings of compartment syndrome may be unreliable, needle compartment pressure monitoring is often useful to evaluate an impending compartment syndrome. In these cases, a ΔP less than 30 mmHg will indicate the possible need for fasciotomy. However, compartment pressure monitoring is not a panacea for challenging clinical scenarios. As demonstrated by Heckman et al., compartment pressures taken from a few centimeters away from fracture site yield unreliable results [15]. One study observing 48 consecutive patients with tibial shaft fractures who were not suspected of developing compartment syndrome underwent pressure measurement of all four lower leg compartments [29]. There was an observed false-positive rate of 35% with the standard threshold of ΔP less than 30 mmHg. Depending upon a single compartment pressure as a sole criteria of surgical intervention would therefore result in unnecessary surgery and morbidity. This reinforces the necessity of clinical observations and judgment that provide context and correct diagnosis compartment syndrome.

Future Directions

The goal of future improvements in the diagnosis of compartment syndrome will obviously focus on increased accuracy, speed, and ease of diagnosis. The current state of practice requires clinical judgment resulting from experience and training. Although the use of pressure monitoring provides a more objective finding, it is a technique that is dependent upon technique and a limited understanding of the threshold of ischemic changes within extremities. Other modalities to better predict and measure intracompartmental pressures will likely improve our ability to diagnose and treat compartment syndrome.

Take-Home Message
The diagnosis and management of suspected compartment syndrome is a troubling situation for any clinician. The risks for long-term morbidity are present even with the most attentive and thorough evaluation. One must be suspicious not only in cases of high-energy trauma and crush injuries but also in unusual circumstances when patients show concerning signs of pressure and pain. The use of compartment pressure monitoring is a useful supplemental tool, but surgeons should be hesitant to base management solely on a single pressure measurement. Clinical judgment and close monitoring are the best tools we have to treat patients presenting with suspected compartment syndrome.

References

1. Seddon HJ. Volkmann's ischaemia in the lower limb. J Bone Joint Surg Br. 1966;48(4):627–36.
2. Owen R, Tsimboukis B. Ischaemia complicating closed tibial and fibular shaft fractures. J Bone Joint Surg Br. 1967;49(2):268–75.
3. O'Toole RV, Whitney A, Merchant N, Hui E, Higgins J, Kim TT, Sagebien C. Variation in diagnosis of compartment syndrome by surgeons treating tibial shaft fractures. J Trauma. 2009;67(4):735–41.
4. Finkelstein JA, Hunter GA, Hu RW. Lower limb compartment syndrome: course after delayed fasciotomy. J Trauma. 1996;40(3):342–4.
5. Sheridan GW, Matsen FA 3rd. Fasciotomy in the treatment of the acute compartment syndrome. J Bone Joint Surg Am. 1976;58(1):112–5.
6. Olson SA, Glasgow RR. Acute compartment syndrome in lower extremity musculoskeletal trauma. J Am Acad Orthop Surg. 2005;13(7):436–44.
7. Ouellette EA. Compartment syndromes in obtunded patients. Hand Clin. 1998;14(3):431–50.
8. Fitzgerald AM, Gaston P, Wilson Y, Quaba A, McQueen MM. Long-term sequelae of fasciotomy wounds. Br J Plast Surg. 2000;53(8):690–3.
9. Velmahos GC, Toutouzas KG. Vascular trauma and compartment syndromes. Surg Clin North Am. 2002;82(1):125–41, xxi.
10. Seddon H. Volkmann's Ischaemia. Br Med J. 1964;1(5398):1587–92.
11. Heckman MM, Whitesides TE Jr, Grewe SR, Judd RL, Miller M, Lawrence JH 3rd. Histologic determination of the ischemic threshold of muscle in the canine compartment syndrome model. J Orthop Trauma. 1993;7(3):199–210.
12. Heppenstall RB, Sapega AA, Izant T, Fallon R, Shenton D, Park YS, Chance B. Compartment syndrome: a quantitative study of high-energy phosphorus compounds using 31P-magnetic resonance spectroscopy. J Trauma. 1989;29(8):1113–9.
13. McQueen MM, Christie J, Court-Brown CM. Acute compartment syndrome in tibial diaphyseal fractures. J Bone Joint Surg Br. 1996;78(1):95–8.
14. Matsen FA 3rd, Winquist RA, Krugmire RB Jr. Diagnosis and management of compartmental syndromes. J Bone Joint Surg Am. 1980;62(2):286–91.
15. Heckman MM, Whitesides TE Jr, Grewe SR, Rooks MD. Compartment pressure in association with closed tibial fractures. The relationship between tissue pressure, compartment, and the distance from the site of the fracture. J Bone Joint Surg Am. 1994;76(9):1285–92.
16. Halpern AA, Nagel DA. Anterior compartment pressures in patients with tibial fractures. J Trauma. 1980;20(9):786–90.
17. Whitesides TE, Heckman MM. Acute compartment syndrome: update on diagnosis and treatment. J Am Acad Orthop Surg. 1996;4(4):209–18.
18. McQueen MM, Gaston P, Court-Brown CM. Acute compartment syndrome. Who is at risk? J Bone Joint Surg Br. 2000;82(2):200–3.
19. Bhattacharyya T, Vrahas MS. The medical-legal aspects of compartment syndrome. J Bone Joint Surg Am. 2004;86-A(4):864–8.
20. DePasse JM, Sargent R, Fantry AJ, Bokshan SL, Palumbo MA, Daniels AH. Assessment of malpractice claims associated with acute compartment syndrome. J Am Acad Orthop Surg. 2017;25(6):e109–13.
21. Harvey EJ, Sanders DW, Shuler MS, Lawendy AR, Cole AL, Alqahtani SM, Schmidt AH. What's new in acute compartment syndrome? J Orthop Trauma. 2012;26(12):699–702.
22. Suk M. I've been served… now what? J Orthop Trauma. 2015;29(Suppl 11):S15–6. https://doi.org/10.1097/BOT.0000000000000436. Review.
23. Jena AB, Seabury S, Lakdawalla D, Chandra A. Malpractice risk according to physician specialty. N Engl J Med. 2011;365(7):629–36.
24. McQueen MM, Court-Brown CM. Compartment monitoring in tibial fractures. The pressure threshold for decompression. J Bone Joint Surg Br. 1996;78(1):99–104.

25. Ulmer T. The clinical diagnosis of compartment syndrome of the lower leg: are clinical findings predictive of the disorder? J Orthop Trauma. 2002;16(8):572–7.
26. Eyres KS, Hill G, Magides A. Compartment syndrome in tibial shaft fracture missed because of a local nerve block. J Bone Joint Surg Br. 1996;78(6):996–7.
27. Mubarak SJ, Wilton NC. Compartment syndromes and epidural analgesia. J Pediatr Orthop. 1997;17(3):282–4.
28. Price C, Ribeiro J, Kinnebrew T. Compartment syndromes associated with postoperative epidural analgesia. A case report. J Bone Joint Surg Am. 1996;78(4):597–9.
29. Whitney A, O'Toole RV, Hui E, Sciadini MF, Pollak AN, Manson TT, Eglseder WA, Andersen RC, Lebrun C, Doro C, Nascone JW. Do one-time intracompartmental pressure measurements have a high false-positive rate in diagnosing compartment syndrome? J Trauma Acute Care Surg. 2014;76(2):479–83.

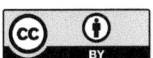

Chapter 2
Legal Aspects of Compartment Syndrome

Milton T. M. Little, Carol A. Lin, and Mark S. Vrahas

> **Objectives**
> - Understand the relationship between malpractice and orthopedic surgery
> - Recognize the medicolegal implications of missed compartment syndrome
> - Understand factors which contribute to indemnity payments with acute compartment syndrome
> - Discuss methods of avoiding compartment syndrome-related litigation

Introduction

Acute compartment syndrome is one of the few orthopedic emergencies requiring urgent evaluation and intervention. The sequelae of missed compartment syndrome include loss of limb, kidney failure, sepsis, and death [1–3]. As such, early evaluation of patients is essential for adequate care and treatment. This chapter will discuss the medicolegal aspects of the treatment of compartment syndrome and its associated complications. There is a paucity of orthopedic research evaluating the factors that lead to malpractice claims and indemnity payments in acute compartment syndrome cases. Despite this, it is essential to thoroughly examine the available data and provide guidelines for the care of these complex patients.

M. T. M. Little (✉)
Cedars-Sinai Medical Center, Orthopedic Surgery Department, Cedars-Sinai Orthopedic Center, Los Angeles, CA, USA
e-mail: Milton.Little@cshs.org

C. A. Lin · M. S. Vrahas
Cedars-Sinai Medical Center, Department of Orthopedic Surgery, Los Angeles, CA, USA

© The Author(s) 2019
C. Mauffrey et al. (eds.), *Compartment Syndrome*,
https://doi.org/10.1007/978-3-030-22331-1_2

The objectives of this chapter are as follows:

1. To understand the relationship between malpractice claims and orthopedic surgery
2. To recognize the medicolegal implications of a missed compartment syndrome
3. To understand the factors that contribute to malpractice claims and indemnity payments
4. To develop a method of patient evaluation to limit the risks of missed compartment syndrome and avoid compartment syndrome-related litigation

Malpractice and Orthopedics

7.6% of all physicians have been named in a malpractice claim in their careers, while 1.6% of physicians have been named in a claim leading to an indemnity payment. Orthopedic surgery is one of top five specialties facing malpractice claims each year [4]. In an analysis of malpractice claims between 1991 and 2005, orthopedic surgeons faced 14% of all malpractice claims during that time period. Neurosurgery was the specialty with the highest number of claims (i.e., 19.1%). The mean indemnity payment for the orthopedic surgery claims has been anywhere from $136,000 to $460,000 [5–7]. For those specialties in the top five, it is estimated that 99% of all physicians will face a malpractice claim by the time they reach the age of 65. Those numbers can lead to significant physician anxiety regarding the risks associated with patient care. Despite the large number of claims, surgeries, and possible outcomes, nearly 75% of the orthopedic malpractice claims rule in favor of the physician [4].

These are a few specific terms to keep in mind when discussing malpractice [8]:

- *Medical negligence*: The breach of duty of care owed by a doctor to a patient that results in damage
- *Standard of care*: The level of care and skill in treatment that, under the circumstances, is recognized as acceptable and appropriate by reasonably prudent similar healthcare providers.
- *Breach of duty*: The doctor fails to work up to the standard of skill required by the law.

Five factors must be present for a malpractice claim to be ruled in favor of the plaintiff:

1. One must prove that a physician-patient relationship existed.
2. There must have been a deviation from the standard of care during the treatment of the patient.
3. The patient must sustain an injury or poor outcome as a result of a deviation from that standard of care.
4. The actions of the physician must be proven to be the cause of the injury [7].

The number of malpractice claims filed per year has continued to rise steadily in Canada, United States, and England [9, 10]. Additionally, significant increases in the sizes of indemnity payments have led to an increased need for malpractice insurance for physicians. One UK hospital found an approximately £40 million increase in payments for negligence between 2006 and 2007 [9].

The increasing number and size of claims has led to increased cost for malpractice insurance which, in turn, has created cyclic crises in the medical field. The United States has faced three serious malpractice crises in the last 50 years [11]. In the 1970s, a crisis availability occurred as an exodus of malpractice insurers became rampant due to the growing numbers of payments. In the 1980s, there was a crisis of affordability as the malpractice insurers increased premiums making them too expensive for some physicians. In the early 2000s, there was a crisis of affordability and availability caused by the departure of several major insurers, leading physicians to turn to prohibitively expensive state-sponsored Joint Underwriting Associations as a last resort. It has been hypothesized that this most recent crisis was caused in part by increased payments, increased frequency of claims, aggressive trial lawyers, and changing public perceptions of medicine in which patients expect perfection [11].

All of these factors have altered the way physicians are treating patients. A survey assessment of orthopedic surgeons showed that 96% of orthopedic surgeons practice defensive medicine by ordering imaging, lab test, and referrals or even admitting patients to the hospital to avoid the risk of a malpractice. Additionally, they reported that approximately 24% of all their tests were ordered as defensive measures and resulted in nearly $2 billion annually [12].

A comparison of the cost between orthopedic trauma surgeons and other subspecialties showed that orthopedic trauma surgeons utilize resources for defensive purposes slightly less than their counterparts (20.3% vs 23%). This comparison still resulted in nearly $7800 per month and $256.3 million per year. Additionally, it was noted that nearly 70% of physicians actually reduced the number of high-risk patients that they accepted into their practice over the last 5 years [13]. It is in this complex climate that we must assess the medicolegal implications compartment syndrome.

Acute Compartment Syndrome and Malpractice

Most analyses of malpractice are performed on closed claims from the state, high volume malpractice insurances, or large-scale databases (national and international). These studies allow one to assess the number of malpractice claims filed for acute compartment syndrome as well as analyze the indemnity payments and the factors leading to the specific ruling in many of the cases. Unfortunately, these closed claim analyses do not provide us with the total number of cases of acute compartment syndrome per year. Therefore, it is difficult to truly assess the risk of facing a malpractice claim in all cases of compartment syndrome. A closed claim analysis performed by Bhattacharyya demonstrated an annual 0.002% claims of practice per orthopedic surgeon [7].

Examination of the defendants in the acute compartment syndrome claims provides some insight into the causes of these claims. When evaluating acute traumatic compartment syndrome, traumatologists were the most commonly named defendants, but when evaluating elective surgery, vascular surgeons (18.2%) were the most commonly sued specialty followed by orthopedists (9.2%) [5]. In one study, orthopedic surgeons were the most common defendants (40.1%) in all claims, followed by nonsurgical providers (38.1%), general surgeons (10.8%), vascular surgeons (6.5%), and plastic surgeons (4.3%) [14]. Understanding the defendants allows us to understand the impact of compartment syndrome on the medical field and how easily one could miss the diagnosis. One must be acutely aware of the signs and symptoms of compartment syndrome in all cases, not just tibia fractures or trauma cases.

Understanding the plaintiffs in these cases is just as critical as understanding the defendants. New York (24.5%) and California (18%) were the locations with the majority of the compartment syndrome claims with Michigan (9.4%) a distant third [5]. Between 20% and 27% of compartment syndrome claims were in pediatric patients, and 27–38% of the claims were in female patients [5, 7, 14]. Men aged 11–30 years old were the highest group of patients presenting with acute compartment syndrome [15]. For patients undergoing elective surgeries, they included total hip/knee arthroplasty, osteotomies, bypass grafts, fistula, abdominal aortic aneurysm repair, skin traction, plastic surgeries, and even "transsexual surgeries." Due to small sample sizes, the frequencies of each were not assessed.

These studies have the unique ability to show us many of the details surrounding acute compartment syndrome claims including the mechanism of injury. DePasse et al. showed that 42.4% of the compartment syndrome cases resulted from acute trauma situations, and surprisingly, 36.75% resulted from elective or cardiac procedures [5]. Marchesi et al. reported an even higher percentage of claims related to acute trauma (63%), with 36% related to elective surgery. More than 70% of acute trauma cases are due to tibia fractures, which is not surprising as it is the most common injury associated with compartment syndrome [5, 7]. Bhataccharya and Vrahas found that 12 of 16 compartment syndrome cases in their report were traumatic tibia fractures, most of which were treated with closed reduction and casting. On the contrary, the majority of thigh compartment syndromes resulted from elective surgery, while the majority of forearm compartment resulted from traumatic injuries (i.e., supracondylar humerus fractures) [5]. Intravenous infiltration (10.1%) is the 3rd most common cause of compartment syndrome claims, and these claims included many nonsurgical hospital staff as defendants.

The signs and symptoms present in the plaintiffs were examined in many of these studies. Between 55% and 68% patients in the cases presented with severe pain as the primary symptom of compartment syndrome [7, 14]. Paresthesias, numbness, or increased compartment tension to palpation were the second common presenting symptoms. Surprisingly, only one study noted the frequency with which compartment pressures were measured, and the frequency was only 25% in their study [7,

14]. Other presenting symptoms included the other cardinal signs of compartment syndrome (e.g., pallor, poikilothermia, paralysis, pulselessness, and pain with passive stretch), but these were less frequently noted [7, 14].

Timing to fasciotomy and sequela of missed compartment were also examined in these closed claims studies. Sixty-eight percent of patients underwent fasciotomies following diagnosis of the symptoms with an average of 3.5 subsequent surgeries [7, 14]. Moreover, 32% of patients underwent delayed fasciotomy (> 8 hours post first sign/symptom) [14], and 18–24% of patients underwent amputations post fasciotomy [5, 7]. Finally, 77% of patients reported permanent physical disability as a result of a missed compartment syndrome [15]. The most common complications were weakness/numbness and contracture in 58% followed by persistent pain, subsequent operations, difficulty walking, and scarring [5].

Delays in diagnosis (87%) and in treatment (36.7%) were the most common causes of acute compartment syndrome claims [5, 7, 14, 15]. This is understandable considering the difficulty in establishing a diagnosis of compartment syndrome. Often, physicians are reluctant to perform compartment pressure measurements due to the level of discomfort they cause to patients. Additionally, the patient's pain may be attributed to postsurgical or post-injury-related pain rather than compartment syndrome. Medications may be utilized to control the pain, leading to masking of the symptoms. Patients who had documented signs such as paresthesias or pain with passive stretch without further investigation were more likely to win the trial or participate in a settled case. Failure to investigate phone calls from patients or disregarding patient complaints without further investigation (poor physician-patient communication) more likely results in ruling for the plaintiff [7]. The studies demonstrated mixed results regarding the impact of patient sex, age, and level of disability with the ruling of the claims and that will be discussed below with the indemnity payments. Based on their report, Bhattacharyya et al. concluded that a fasciotomy within 8 hours of presentation and early action once physical findings are documented could prevent a malpractice claim [7].

The plaintiffs were successful in 56–77% of the claims in the studies examined [5, 7, 14, 15] with 27–56% of the claims resulting in a settlement rather than trial [5, 7]. Depasse et al. reported that 68% of trials were won by the defendant, and the Bhattacharyya study reported that the defendant was successful in all three cases that went to trial [5, 7]. Marchesi found that 72% of the damages were due to the physician's actions or inaction [14]. Interestingly, the post procedure compartment syndrome was more commonly ruled in favor of the plaintiffs compared to traumatic compartment syndrome where the sequelae were thought to be due to the injuries themselves rather than the physicians. Depasse et al. reported that cases with pediatric plaintiffs were more likely to be settled out of court and that judges were more likely to rule in favor of pediatric plaintiffs than adult plaintiffs. Additionally, they also demonstrated that judges were more likely to rule in favor of female plaintiffs than male plaintiffs. There was no sex or age-related differences in indemnity payments in the studies [5].

The indemnity payments in the acute compartment syndrome cases far exceed the average indemnity payment ($136,000) for orthopedic surgeons' malpractice claims. Cases that were settled reported indemnity payments from $52,500 to $3,500,000, whereas cases that went to court reported indemnity payments from $106,970 to $22,565,000 [5]. Indemnity payments were noted to correlate linearly with the number of presenting cardinal signs of compartment syndrome as well as with the time to fasciotomy [7]. The indemnity payments were significantly higher in the post procedure acute compartment syndrome (mean $3,399,035) compared to the traumatic compartment syndrome ($986,716) [5]. There was no significant difference in the indemnity payments for juvenile or female patients when compared to their adult or male counterparts. And there was no association between amputation or level of dysfunction and indemnity payment.

Patient Assessment and Future Directions

The sequela and medicolegal ramifications of missed compartment syndrome are severe. Training institutions in particular face unique difficulties with the implementation of the 80-hour work week. Limitations in staffing necessitate an increased number of patient handoffs which can lead to poor physician communication, lack of care coordination and continuity, and an increased likelihood of missed diagnoses [2]. As noted above, delay in diagnosis and delay in intervention are the most common causes of malpractice claims in acute compartment syndrome cases. Developing a systematic approach to patient care is critical to avoiding malpractice claims, indemnity payments, and poor patient outcomes. Garner et al. described an algorithm for care of patients at risk for compartment syndrome which we review below [2].

The first step in the care of these patients is recognizing who are at high risk for development of compartment syndrome, most commonly victims of trauma (tibia fractures, supracondylar humerus fractures, and crush injuries). It is also essential to recognize that patients outside of these categories may also develop compartment syndrome (vascular bypass, IV infiltration, elective procedures and plastic surgery). These high-risk patients should be assessed by the oncoming team and the outgoing team together to compare the examination findings and medication administration record. Careful communication pre- and postoperatively should be performed with the patients regarding the signs and risks of compartment syndrome. Patients or their families should be informed of the sequelae of a missed compartment syndrome as well as the clinical course of those patients diagnosed and treated for compartment syndrome. In particular, the limb-saving nature of fasciotomies for this condition should be emphasized. This communication is critical for the patient to have appropriate expectations regarding the condition, the necessity of treatment, and the possible need for additional interventions.

Patients should be assessed closely for increasing analgesic requirements and any of the cardinal signs or symptoms of compartment syndrome with worsening pain aggravated by passive muscle stretch being the essential sign [16]. Increasing medication requirements may be the only sign of a nascent compartment syndrome in young children or patients who have difficulties in communicating. Paresthesias and severe pain should be investigated fully by opening splints/dressings and close monitoring for any improvement or changes. After discussing with senior staffing, there should be a low threshold for compartment pressure measurements in any patient displaying any of the cardinal signs. While palpation of compartments is the most commonly reported aspect of the exam, it has been shown to have a very poor correlation with a true diagnosis of compartment syndrome with reported sensitivities as low as 24% [17].

Patients should be examined by the same medical professional every 2–4 hours until the combined pass-on examination between staff members. Care must be taken in obtunded patients or patients who have undergone regional analgesia or neuraxial block pre or post procedure as the symptoms may be masked. The threshold for compartment measurements should be even lower in these patients. However, while intra-compartmental pressures have a high estimated sensitivity and specificity, it is still possible to have both false-positive and false-negative results, and so the patient's clinical presentation should be heavily considered. Though fasciotomies can be morbid procedures, many consider the significant sequelae of untreated compartment syndrome to be worse. As such, surgeons can expect that up to 3–4% of clinically concerning patients undergoing fasciotomies may not ultimately have a true compartment syndrome so as to be certain that no cases are ever missed [18].

Take-Home Messages
- Compartment syndrome accounts for 0.03–0.05% of all malpractice claims per year.
- Misdiagnosed compartment syndrome and delayed compartment releases result in some of the highest indemnity payments in orthopedic litigation.
- Compartment syndrome following elective surgery, female sex, young plaintiffs, and the presence of cardinal symptoms (pain out of proportion, paresthesias, pallor, poikilothermia, pulselessness) is associated with a high rate of plaintiff victory in litigation.
- Thorough documentation, early compartment releases (<8 hours), and clear physician-patient communication decrease the risk of plaintiff victory in compartment syndrome litigation.
- Consistent examination and early action when symptoms develop are critical to properly diagnose compartment syndrome.

Bibliography

1. Taylor RM, Sullivan MP, Mehta S. Acute compartment syndrome: obtaining diagnosis, providing treatment, and minimizing medicolegal risk. Curr Rev Musculoskelet Med. 2012;5(3):206–13.

 2. Garner MR, Taylor SA, Gausden E, Lyden JP. Compartment syndrome: diagnosis, management, and unique concerns in the twenty-first century. HSS J. 2014;10(2):143–52.
 3. Elliott KGB, Johnstone AJ. Diagnosing acute compartment syndrome. J Bone Joint Surg. 2003;85-B(5):625–32.
 4. Jena AB, Seabury S, Lakdawalla D, Chandra A. Malpractice risk according to physician specialty. N Engl J Med. 2011;365(7):629–36.
 5. DePasse JM, Sargent R, Fantry AJ, Bokshan SL, Palumbo MA, Daniels AH. Assessment of malpractice claims associated with acute compartment syndrome. J Am Acad Orthop Surg. 2017;25(6):e109–e13.
 6. Liability CoP. Managing Orthopaedic Malpractice Risk. 2nd ed. Rosemont: American Academy of Orthopaedic Surgeons; 2000.
 7. Bhattacharyya T, Vrahas MS. The medical-legal aspects of compartment syndrome. J Bone Joint Surg Am. 2004;86-A(4):864–8.
 8. Thomas TG. Orthopaedic manholes and rabbit holes- some thoughts on medical negligence. J R Soc Med. 1986;79(12):701–7.
 9. Atrey A, Gupte CM, Corbett SA. Review of successful litigation against english health trusts in the treatment of adults with orthopaedic pathology: clinical governance lessons learned. J Bone Joint Surg Am. 2010;92(18):e36.
10. Gidwani S, Zaidi SM, Bircher MD. Medical negligence in orthopaedic surgery: a review of 130 consecutive medical negligence reports. J Bone Joint Surg Br. 2009;91(2):151–6.
11. Mello MM, Studdert DM, Brennan TA. The new medical malpractice crisis. N Engl J Med. 2003;348(23):2281–4.
12. Sethi MK, Obremskey W, Natividad H, Mir HR, Jahangir AA. Incidence and costs of defensive medicine among orthopedic surgeons in the United States: a national survey study. Am J Orthop. 2012;41(2):69–73.
13. Sathiyakumar V, Jahangir AA, Mir HR, Obremskey WT, Lee YM, Apfeld JC, et al. The prevalence and costs of defensive medicine among orthopaedic trauma surgeons: a national survey study. J Orthop Trauma. 2013;27(10):592–7.
14. Marchesi M, Marchesi A, Calori GM, Cireni LV, Sileo G, Merzagora I, et al. A sneaky surgical emergency: acute compartment syndrome. Retrospective analysis of 66 closed claims, medico-legal pitfalls and damages evaluation. Injury. 2014;45(Suppl 6):S16–20.
15. Shadgan BMM, Sanders D, Berry G, Martin C Jr, Duffy P, Stephen D, O'Brien PJ. Current thinking about acute compartment syndrome of the lower extremity. Can J Surg. 2010;53(5):329–34.
16. Pearse MF, Harry L, Nanchahal J. Acute compartment syndrome of the leg. BMJ. 2002;325(7364):557–8.
17. Shuler FD, Dietz MJ. Physicians' ability to manually detect isolated elevations in leg intracompartmental pressure. J Bone Joint Surg Am. 2010;92(2):361–7.
18. McQueen MM, Duckworth AD, Aitken SA, Court-Brown CM. The estimated sensitivity and specificity of compartment pressure monitoring for acute compartment syndrome. J Bone Joint Surg Am. 2013;95(8):673–7.

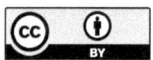

Chapter 3
Pathophysiology of Compartment Syndrome

Geraldine Merle and Edward J. Harvey

Background

- Pathophysiology stems from pressure-related changes in the affected muscle.
- Exact mechanisms are not clearly understood, but some models have been postulated.
- Local pressure phenomena and reperfusion injury account for the clinical issues.
- Diagnosis has been inaccurate which has impeded the full understanding of pathophysiology.

Inciting Factors in Early Compartment Syndrome

Traditional teaching is that acute compartment syndrome (ACS) occurs when locally increased tissue pressure compromises local circulation and neuromuscular function [1–5]. Circulatory patency is what maintains normal tissue function in the affected tissues including importantly nerves and muscles. Functional abnormality results after initiation of factors leading to ACS. Several markers of ACS have been used or sought and are currently seen as a direct result of the pathophysiology changes not as initiating factors. Trauma to the area results in swelling, ischemia, inflammation, patchy oxygen metabolism deficiencies, and increasing pressure [5, 6]. The question of which of these pathological changes comes first in the ACS

G. Merle
Montreal General Hospital, Montreal, QC, Canada
e-mail: geraldine.merle@mcgill.ca

E. J. Harvey (✉)
McGill University, Michal and Renata Hornstein Chair in Surgical Excellence, Montreal General Hospital, Montreal, QC, Canada
e-mail: edward.harvey@mcgill.ca

© The Author(s) 2019
C. Mauffrey et al. (eds.), *Compartment Syndrome*,
https://doi.org/10.1007/978-3-030-22331-1_3

scenario is a little like the chicken or the egg debate in that it may not be as important as the actual diagnosis. Hargens et al. [7] found normal capillary pressure to be between 20 and 33 mm Hg. Pressures above this have been deemed sufficient to shut off flow and cause ischemia. Normal interstitial fluid pressure is around 10 mmHg, a value fairly close to the capillary pressure. Authors [8] initially observed that with progressively higher applied external pressures, the blood flow to that area ceased before the difference between mean arterial and applied pressure became zero. This was the basis of the critical closure theory. A significant transmural pressure is theorized to maintain arteriolar patency. Tension in the walls of arterioles is actively produced by smooth muscle contraction. If tissue pressure is elevated enough, transmural pressure is insufficient for the arterioles to actively close and blood flow is arrested [9]. Support for critical closure was further gained from the studies of Ashton [8] on the effect of limb temperature. It was demonstrated that the critical transmural pressure varied with limb temperature in that a greater transmural pressure was required to maintain blood flow when local cooling increased the tone of arteriolar wall smooth muscle. Would critical closure be sufficient for prolonged compartmental ischemia? Ischemia causes vasodilation, which may bring more fluid into the affected compartment. Undoubtedly, this theory could be consistent with early ACS but probably does not explain ACS propagation in borderline cases. Other authors [10, 11] have discussed increases in tissue pressure being responsible for reduction in the local arteriovenous gradient and thereby local blood flow. When the metabolic demands of the tissue are insufficiently met by reduced flow from increased pressure, a compartmental syndrome may result. This theory does not dictate a zero-flow scenario and is therefore more reasonable and is a better model of ACS.

All of the factors that change the metabolism of the traumatic zone combined with anatomic limitations in blood supply, muscle fascial covering, and altered physiology result in ACS. Without a doubt the pressure increase is what is best understood as a pathological event or marker by care providers. Increased tissue pressure that compromises local circulation has been demonstrated by many researchers. The method of ascertaining this has changed over the years but has consistently showed that abnormally high pressures are present early in ACS [1, 2, 4–6, 12–19]. The pressure changes the ability of the local circulation to deliver oxygen to the tissue. Monitoring muscle PO_2 has shown the balance between tissue oxygen delivery and tissue oxygen consumption [3, 5, 15–17]. Each zone of the affected area may have a slightly different PO_2 in the initial stages of ACS. With increased swelling and pressure, the whole compartment begins to show the effects. No critical pressure has been observed as a magic tipping point where ACS is definite, and in fact some studies have shown compromise at pressure of 20 mmHg – lower than the currently held trigger point for surgery [10]. The disease process is just a spectrum of pressure changes where there is a greater compromise of muscle PO_2 at higher tissue pressures. There are several proposed mechanisms of pressure-induced circulatory compromise. These include a starling resistor model for flow cessation, irreversible damage to small vessels, clotting mechanisms, and others.

None of these models have really been shown to be the sole mechanism although pressure changes cause most of what is seen physiologically in the early stages.

Most investigators believed that the physiological changes were all pressure related. Sheridan et al. [20] inflated a latex balloon in a muscle compartment of a rabbit. They were looking at the response of nerve and muscle to the added pressure. The PO_2 declined with increasing pressure from an initial control value of about 10 mmHg to a low of 2.8 mmHg at a compartment pressure of 90 mmHg. The integrity of the peroneal nerve and muscles was tested by direct electrical stimulation. Higher pressures and longer periods of pressure application produced more frequent functional losses. In the end, the authors felt that the pressure alone was a sufficient explanation for all changes seen in ACS. Increased tissue pressure also directly compromises neuromuscular function. Rorabeck and Clark [6] and Hargens et al. [7] slowed nerve conduction velocity by the pressurized infusion of the anterior leg compartment of dogs. In general, increased tissue pressure as low as 20 mm Hg affects tissue flow, and tissue circulation is decreased as the applied pressure is raised.

Vollmar et al. were interested in the microvascular response to similar external pressure elevation seen in ACS [21]. They used a skinfold model that was not an exact substitute for a compartment but illustrated a potential physiological change in tissue flow. They studied the response of the different segments of the microcirculation in terms of vasomotor control (change of vessel diameter) and cessation of blood flow with progressive changes in external tissue pressure. They felt that the study disproved the critical closing theory but complied with the hypothesis of reduced arteriovenous pressure gradients as the cause of blood flow decrease in compartment syndrome. They found that there was an increased perfusion pressure gradient needed in order to restart blood flow in small vessels. It was seen as a confirmation of the existence of so-called yield stress in microvessels. The high susceptibility of capillaries to elevated external pressure indicated to the authors that there was a need for early fasciotomy to restore impaired circulation. Lack of effective circulation is the factor that perpetuates further physiological changes and propagates a full compartment syndrome. It is the tipping point of the syndrome. The amount of pressure the muscles can tolerate before deficits are produced is also altered by local blood flow changes with examples being limb elevation, arterial occlusion, hypotension, or hemorrhage [10]. Dilation in the arteriole system caused by injury, along with collapsing smaller vessels and increased permeability, leads to increased fluid extravasation and raised interstitial fluid pressure. As it increases, perfusion to tissue becomes decreased. Once perfusion reaches a low level, tissue hypoxemia results. The combination of hypoxia, increase in oxidant stress, and development of hypoglycemia in the compartmental tissue causes cell edema due to a shutdown of the ATPase channels that maintain cellular osmotic balance [22]. Early ACS microvascular dysfunction results in a decrease in capillary perfusion and an increase in cellular injury and was associated with a severe acute inflammatory component [23]. The loss of cell-membrane potential results in an influx of chloride ions, leading to cellular swelling and ongoing cellular necrosis. The increase in tissue swelling worsens the hypoxic state and creates an ongoing positive feedback. As the cascade of elevated pressure then compromises the microcirculation with decreased oxygen and nutrient delivery, tissue anoxia with eventual myonecrosis then proceeds. In fact, systemic changes have been reported [24] as remote changes in liver and kidney function.

Changing Tissue Tolerance with Increased Pressure

Ongoing pressure and the tissue response are difficult to quantify. Tissues will react in different ways depending on the metabolic demands of the tissue and the duration of the increased pressure. This brings into play the specific effect of increased tissue pressure on local blood flow in the tissues. Bone will react differently than muscle and nerve – the more commonly injured tissues. Nerve and muscle do have a potential for recovery and reconstruction following ischemic injury. Hypotension, hemorrhage, arterial blood flow cessation, and limb elevation all reduce the tolerance of limbs for increased pressure [10]. Hargens et al. [7] elevated tissue pressure by the infusion of autologous plasma. They found some slowing of nerve conduction with a pressure of 30–40 mm Hg for 8–14 hours, but these conditions did not completely arrest nerve conduction. Pressure of 50 mm Hg for 330 minutes did stop nerve conduction. Sheridan et al. [20] inflated a leg balloon in rabbits to investigate the response of nerve and muscle to direct stimulation. Applied pressure of 60 mm Hg for 6 hours produced consistent functional losses. A pressure of 100 mm Hg for 12 hours caused a loss of all nerve or muscle stimulation response. Rorabeck and Clarke [6] found that 40 mm Hg reduced peroneal nerve conduction velocity from 40 to 30 m/sec over 2.5 hours. A pressure of 80 mm Hg arrested peroneal nerve conduction after 4 hours. Certainly, there is a difference amongst subjects and species for tolerance of pressure before nerve conduction slows or stops. There are no studies in the literature on muscle function after pressure initiation. Some researchers have looked at muscle degeneration after ACS conditions. Hargens et al. [7] investigated the effects of increased pressure in their model system using technetium-99 m stannous pyrophosphate. They found that pressures exceeding 20 mm Hg produced in a canine model a significant uptake of the label when maintained for 8 hours. From this point, the amount of uptake increased dramatically as higher pressures were applied. Rorabeck [6] found that when a pressure of 40 mm Hg was applied in a canine model, there was an increased in venous creatinine phosphokinase activity. Similar findings were noted for lactic dehydrogenase. They could not quantify the amount of marker with the amount of pressure applied. This may indicate that there is no hard-critical pressure in every situation or person. If we look at the hypothesis of reduced arteriovenous pressure gradients as the cause of flow cessation in compartment syndrome, then it explains that lower arterial pressure will decrease the pressure tolerance of tissue [10]. Hypotension from halothane anesthetic used for surgery over a 5-hour period was studied. The results showed that the circulatory effect of 60 mm Hg of compartmental pressure was much more apparent in the hypotensive animals. Zweifach [25] also investigated the effects on the pressure tolerance of rabbit limbs after an acute systemic hemorrhage of 20% of blood volume. Applied pressure of 40 mm Hg led to significantly greater reductions in nitrogen washout, muscle oxygenation, and action potentials in the hemorrhage group. They had seen similar results in a canine model. Limb elevation can reduce local arterial pressure; however, elevation alone cannot lower the limb's venous pressure below the level of the local tissue pressure – that in the compartment. Thus for any given tissue pressure elevation of a limb above the supine position, there is a reduction in the local arteriovenous gradient. This means that a lower pressure is paradoxically sufficient to cause damage in an elevated limb [10]. This result of the arteriovenous gradient effect is clinically relevant in that it suggests that limbs with compartments showing signs of inadequate blood flow should not be elevated. Elevation will lower local arterial pressure but will not affect local venous pressure. ACS will evolve quicker than in non-elevated limbs.

Tissue Reperfusion as a Late Inciting Factor for Compartment Syndrome

Necrosis of compartment contents due to low oxygen and nutrient levels does occur eventually with prolonged high pressures. However, another mechanism for ACS propagation does take place with incomplete arterial occlusion or returning perfusion after ischemia. Reperfusion injury is tissue damage caused when blood supply returns to the compartment contents after a period of ischemia [26]. The absence of oxygen and nutrients during ischemia creates an environment whereby restoration of blood flow results in inflammation and oxidative damage rather than complete restoration of normal function [23]. This may occur after reperfusion but must also occur in the period of time where the microenvironment is fluctuating between flow and no-flow conditions at the cellular level. Normal microvascular perfusion is made up of mostly continuously perfused capillaries. Elevated compartment pressure results in a shift of perfusion toward intermittently perfused and non-perfused capillaries [21, 23, 27, 28], leading to low flow ischemic muscle areas. The metabolic demands of the tissue cannot be met, resulting in the production of reactive oxygen species and other inflammatory intermediaries [23]. During ischemia, there is a gradual depletion of intracellular stores of energy. There is a buildup of products of low oxygen metabolism, particularly lactic acid, with accompanying hydrogen ion accumulation [29]. Eventual cellular death occurs in some areas of the compartment. Unlike a complete reperfusion cycle, the defined phases of compartment content injury cannot be clearly delineated in low-flow ischemia. The reperfusion injury would not only persist throughout the duration of the ACS, but would be further intensified by surgical treatment that allows restoration of normal blood flow into the capillary bed. Reperfusion may cause harmful effects by washing out necessary precursors for energy formation. Production of oxygen free radicals and calcium influx both occur with disruption of oxidative rephosphorylation at the mitochondria level [23, 30]. Upregulation of neutrophil receptors and endothelial leucocyte adhesion molecules lead to the sequestration of white blood cells in the muscle (with a prolonged inflammatory response) with prolongation of the reperfusion injury. Capillary endothelium is also damaged by prolonged ischemia with a resultant increase in capillary permeability. Returning perfusion results in extravasation through the damaged areas with an increase in compartment volume. Lawendy et al. [24] demonstrated a two-hit inflammatory model with ACS and fasciotomy representing two hits of the systemic physiology. ACS causes a significant initial rise in the level of TNF-α and is followed by a second peak in the systemic levels of TNF-α after fasciotomy. The second peak is felt to be due to cellular debris, proinflammatory mediators, and cytokines gaining access to the systemic circulation leading to a systemic inflammatory response. Several cytokines are significantly elevated after a few hours of ICP elevation – TNF-α, IL-1β, GRO/KC, MCP-1, MIP-1α, and IL-1 – almost all of which are inflammatory [31]. Continued seeping fluid from damaged capillaries and muscle will only propagate the cascade that results in complete compartment syndrome.

The combination of multiple factors culminates in ACS. Ongoing changes at the cellular level represent early pressure-induced reversible ACS. The vacillating flow-no-flow scenario at the muscle level either causes limited local cellular death and changes or progresses through to complete ACS and more apparent clinical changes. This is microenvironment reperfusion injury propagation. The model of arteriovenous gradient as an explanation for ACS may be close to the truth. Our treatment for ACS results in a more compete reperfusion injury particularly when diagnosis is late. In summary, although many reasons for ACS have been suggested, the main marker for pathophysiological changes remains pressure in the early stages of the syndrome. Continued physiological changes later in the disease can be tracked by other markers in combination with pressure.

Take-Home Message
- Sequelae of high local pressures in a muscle compartment is the main problem.
- Several mechanisms have been postulated with arteriovenous gradient model being most realistic to clinical scenario.
- Pressure interacts with local tissue compromise and changes the resistance to injury.
- Inflammatory mediators and metabolites potentiate the reperfusion injury.

References

1. Matsen FA 3rd, Mayo KA, Sheridan GW, Krugmire RB Jr. Monitoring of intramuscular pressure. Surgery. 1976;79(6):702–9.
2. Rorabeck CH, Bourne RB, Fowler PJ, Finlay JB, Nott L. The role of tissue pressure measurement in diagnosing chronic anterior compartment syndrome. Am J Sports Med. 1988;16(2):143–6.

3. Hansen EN, Manzano G, Kandemir U, Mok JM. Comparison of tissue oxygenation and compartment pressure following tibia fracture. Injury. 2013;44(8):1076–80.
4. Prayson MJ, Chen JL, Hampers D, Vogt M, Fenwick J, Meredick R. Baseline compartment pressure measurements in isolated lower extremity fractures without clinical compartment syndrome. J Trauma. 2006;60(5):1037–40.
5. Clayton JM, Hayes AC, Barnes RW. Tissue pressure and perfusion in the compartment syndrome. J Surg Res. 1977;22(4):333–9.
6. Rorabeck CH, Clarke KM. The pathophysiology of the anterior tibial compartment syndrome: an experimental investigation. J Trauma. 1978;18(5):299–304.
7. Hargens AR, Mubarak SJ. Current concepts in the pathophysiology, evaluation, and diagnosis of compartment syndrome. Hand Clin. 1998;14(3):371–83.
8. Ashton H. The effect of increased tissue pressure on blood flow. Clin Orthop Relat Res. 1975;113:15–26.
9. Pittman R. Oxygen transport in the microcirculation and its regulation. Microcirculation. 2013;20(Feb 2):117–37.
10. Matsen FA 3rd, Wyss CR, King RV, Barnes D, Simmons CW. Factors affecting the tolerance of muscle circulation and function for increased tissue pressure. Clin Orthop Relat Res. 1981;155:224–30.
11. Reneman RS. The anterior and the lateral compartmental syndrome of the leg due to intensive use of muscles. Clin Orthop Relat Res. 1975;113:69–80.
12. Schmidt AH. Acute compartment syndrome. Injury. 2017;48(Suppl 1):S22–S5.
13. Martinez AP, Moser TP, Saran N, Paquet M, Hemmerling T, Berry GK. Phonomyography as a non-invasive continuous monitoring technique for muscle ischemia in an experimental model of acute compartment syndrome. Injury. 2017;48(11):2411–6.
14. Whitney A, O'Toole RV, Hui E, Sciadini MF, Pollak AN, Manson TT, et al. Do one-time intra-compartmental pressure measurements have a high false-positive rate in diagnosing compartment syndrome? J Trauma Acute Care Surg. 2014;76(2):479–83.
15. Garner MR, Taylor SA, Gausden E, Lyden JP. Compartment syndrome: diagnosis, management, and unique concerns in the twenty-first century. HSS J. 2014;10(2):143–52.
16. Harvey EJ, Sanders DW, Shuler MS, Lawendy AR, Cole AL, Alqahtani SM, et al. What's new in acute compartment syndrome? J Orthop Trauma. 2012;26(12):699–702.
17. Ozkayin N, Aktuglu K. Absolute compartment pressure versus differential pressure for the diagnosis of compartment syndrome in tibial fractures. Int Orthop. 2005;29(6):396–401.
18. Kumar P, Salil B, Bhaskara KG, Agrawal A. Compartment syndrome: effect of limb position on pressure measurement. Burns. 2003;29(6):626.
19. Dahn I, Lassen NA, Westling H. Blood flow in human muscles during external pressure or venous stasis. Clin Sci. 1967;32(3):467–73.
20. Sheridan GW, Matsen FA 3rd, Krugmire RB Jr. Further investigations on the pathophysiology of the compartmental syndrome. Clin Orthop Relat Res. 1977;123:266–70.
21. Vollmar B, Westermann S, Menger MD. Microvascular response to compartment syndrome-like external pressure elevation: an in vivo fluorescence microscopic study in the hamster striated muscle. J Trauma. 1999;46(1):91–6.
22. von Keudell AG, Weaver MJ, Appleton PT, Bae DS, Dyer GSM, Heng M, et al. Diagnosis and treatment of acute extremity compartment syndrome. Lancet. 2015;386(10000):1299–310.
23. Lawendy AR, Sanders DW, Bihari A, Parry N, Gray D, Badhwar A. Compartment syndrome-induced microvascular dysfunction: an experimental rodent model. Can J Surg. 2011;54(3):194–200.
24. Lawendy AR, Bihari A, Sanders DW, Badhwar A, Cepinskas G. Compartment syndrome causes systemic inflammation in a rat. Bone Joint J. 2016;98-B(8):1132–7.
25. Zweifach SS, Hargens AR, Evans KL, Smith RK, Mubarak SJ, Akeson WH. Skeletal muscle necrosis in pressurized compartments associated with hemorrhagic hypotension. J Trauma. 1980;20(11):941–7.
26. Perry MO. Compartment syndromes and reperfusion injury. Surg Clin N Am. 1988;68(4):853–64.

27. Owen CA, Mubarak SJ, Hargens AR, Rutherford L, Garetto LP, Akeson WH. Intramuscular pressures with limb compression. Clarification of the pathogenesis of the drug-induced muscle-compartment syndrome. N Engl J Med. 1979;300(21):1169–72.
28. Tollens T, Janzing H, Broos P. The pathophysiology of the acute compartment syndrome. Acta Chir Belg. 1998;98(4):171–5.
29. Caty MG, Guice KS, Oldham KT, Remick DG, Kunkel SI. Evidence for tumor necrosis factor-induced pulmonary microvascular injury after intestinal ischemia-reperfusion injury. Ann Surg. 1990;212(6):694–700.
30. Hartmann P, Eros G, Varga R, Kaszaki J, Garab D, Nemeth I, et al. Limb ischemia-reperfusion differentially affects the periosteal and synovial microcirculation. J Surg Res. 2012;178(1):216–22.
31. Ascer E, Gennaro M, Cupo S, Mohan C. Do cytokines play a role in skeletal muscle ischemia and reperfusion? J Cardiovasc Surg. 1992;33(5):588–92.

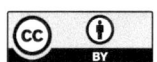

Chapter 4
Determining Ischaemic Thresholds Through Our Understanding of Cellular Metabolism

Alan J. Johnstone and Derek Ball

Background to the Chapter

- Synopsis of clinical issues associated with the complexity of compartment syndromes and current diagnostic limitations
- Comprehending the metabolic capacity of active skeletal muscle and its constant need for energy
- Understanding the principle of an ischaemic threshold and the localised techniques that are employed by muscle to counteract progressive ischaemia
- Investigating the potential for tissue concentrations of key biochemical molecules involved in aerobic and anaerobic respiration to become markers of ischaemia
- Investigating the role of direct tissue pH monitoring to become a future objective measure of muscle metabolic status related to ischaemia irrespective of the cause

Clinical Issues and Concerns

Compartment syndromes, through their definition, are complex, multifactorial and ultimately result in irreversible cell damage leading to cell death. Although their causation differs, influenced significantly by a number of local or systemic factors,

A. J. Johnstone (✉)
Aberdeen Royal Infirmary & University of Aberdeen, Orthopedic Trauma Unit,
Aberdeen, Grampian Region, UK
e-mail: alan.johnstone@abdn.ac.uk

D. Ball
School of Medicine, University of Aberdeen, Medical Sciences and Nutrition,
Aberdeen, Aberdeenshire, UK
e-mail: derek.ball@abdn.ac.uk

© The Author(s) 2019
C. Mauffrey et al. (eds.), *Compartment Syndrome*,
https://doi.org/10.1007/978-3-030-22331-1_4

they all have one thing in common – progressive tissue ischaemia that if unchecked results in death of the cells within the affected limb [1]. The most widely studied and understood form of compartment syndrome is trauma-related compartment syndrome, often referred to as acute compartment syndrome (ACS) and can occur following fractures, soft tissue crush injuries or burns. However, clinicians should also be aware of the significant effects that systemic hypotension or hypoxia can have upon an injured limb that is already compromised, has a higher metabolic need compared with uninjured tissues and is therefore prone to develop this otherwise insidious complication.

With particular reference to ACS, accurately diagnosing this syndrome remains a challenge since the clinical symptoms and signs that accompany early-stage ACS are difficult to differentiate from those that accompany the original injury, and for this reason, there has been considerable interest in developing objective tests that could aid diagnosis and permit earlier intervention resulting in better long-term clinical outcomes. The most commonly used objective method for diagnosing ACS is to measure intracompartmental pressure (ICP) [2] since trauma results in localised swelling that in turn gives rise to an increase in the ICP, which undoubtedly contributes to the underlying soft tissue ischaemia. However, despite the wide acceptance of Matsen's arteriovenous gradient theory behind the pathophysiology of ACS, which elegantly explains the mechanical aspects of this syndrome, it lacks useful information about the underlying cellular effects especially in the presence of injury and the resultant increase in requirements for energy by the injured cells. Overall, the majority of clinicians remain unconvinced about the value of monitoring ICP given its well-documented poor diagnostic specificity, and the search continues for better objective diagnostic methods [3].

Skeletal Muscle Physiology

Skeletal muscle is a highly metabolically active tissue. Even at rest, it has been calculated that the turnover of adenosine triphosphate (ATP) is around 35 μmol.kg^{-1} muscle, with the energy used mainly to transport Ca^{2+} and to maintain the balance of intracellular and extracellular Na^+ and K^+ across the sarcolemma [4]. However, skeletal muscle can rapidly increase its consumption of ATP by approximately 1000-fold (5 mmol.kg^{-1}) during maximum exercise with 70% of the ATP being utilised to undertake muscular work through the interaction of myosin and actin and the remaining 30% employed to transport Ca^{2+}, Na^+ and K^+ [5]. There is a very limited store of ATP resulting in a constant requirement for ATP to be replenished. When oxygen delivery and availability is abundant, ATP is primarily re-synthesised through oxidative phosphorylation of fatty acids via mitochondrial respiration, but during periods of increased energy turnover, glycogen and glucose are also used as substrates to produce ATP. This process is also known as aerobic respiration. However, when oxygen availability and/or delivery is below that required for oxidative phosphorylation, the energy required to re-synthesise ATP is produced through glycolysis (also known as anaerobic respiration); under these circumstances, the end product of glycolysis, pyruvate, is converted to lactic acid, resulting in an accumulation of H^+ ions intra- and extracellularly. After high-intensity exercise, the metabolic consequence is that intramuscular pH levels can be as low as 6.5 [6]. Although in the liver, lactate can be oxidised to pyruvate and ultimately converted into glucose-6-phosphate which can then be utilised for oxidative phosphorylation. Since the enzymes required for this conversion are not present in the skeletal muscle, lactic acid could be considered a metabolically 'dead end' molecule in muscle and only becomes a useful source of energy when it is transported to the liver where it is reprocessed through gluconeogenesis [7]. To exacerbate matters, given that ACS results in a gradual reduction of venous blood flow, the mechanism for reprocessing of lactate by the liver becomes increasingly restricted resulting in an accelerated build-up of lactic acid within muscle. The H^+ ions that accumulate intracellularly, as a result of anaerobic respiration, are buffered to some degree by intracellular proteins, although a sizeable proportion are actively transported extracellularly where they can be buffered by plasma bicarbonate and the lactic acid used in the liver as a substrate through gluconeogenesis.

In extreme circumstances when the muscles' need for energy is exceptionally high and glycolysis is insufficient, the high-energy phosphate-containing molecules, phosphocreatine (PCr) and adenosine diphosphate (ADP), can be catabolised [8]. However, this process results in a reduction in the total adenine nucleotide pool [9], a situation that is still reversible but requires considerable future energy reserves to rectify and resembles a pre-terminal stage for the cell.

When Reversible Cell Injury Becomes Irreversible

Cells are remarkably tolerant to ischaemia, but in the absence of sufficient energy reserves, cell membrane ion exchange pumps become less efficient resulting in an accumulation of Na^+ intracellularly and a diffusion of K^+ out of the cells features that are associated with cellular swelling; overall protein synthesis slows; and in muscle there is reduced contractility. However, if the delivery of adequately oxygenated blood is restored, all of these cellular disturbances are reversible.

Irreversible injury is associated with morphological features such as severe swelling of mitochondria, extensive damage to plasma membranes and swelling of lysosomes. These features result in mitochondria that are unable to synthesise ATP and plasma and organelle membrane damage that leads to structural loss of the cell and the organelles resulting in the undesirable entry of extracellular proteins and loss of intracellular proteins. It is at this stage that myocyte specific proteins such as troponin and creatine kinase are released into the extracellular fluid and are useful blood biomarkers of cellular damage. Loss of membrane integrity also results in extracellular Ca^{2+} entering the cell and in particular the mitochondria. In circumstances where the irreversibly damaged cells are reperfused, Ca^{2+} is taken up rapidly by the mitochondria and permanently poisons them through inhibiting enzyme activity. Also, oxygen free radicals are produced on restoration of the blood supply resulting in further direct injury to the plasma and organelle membranes.

In summary, membrane injury and subsequent significant dysfunction is the central factor leading to irreversible cell injury.

Coping Mechanisms That Are Employed by Skeletal Muscle in Response to Ischaemia

Hypo-perfusion resulting in localised ischaemia is a fact of everyday life, where cells, tissues and organs are perpetually utilising a variety of coping mechanisms to promote blood flow, varying oxygen extraction from the blood, and to modify cellular metabolism to generate energy depending upon the concentration of oxygen that is locally available.

1. Autoregulation is the term given to the ability of the microcirculation to reduce vascular resistance through relaxing the smooth muscle present within the vessel walls that in turn improves blood flow in situations when the arteriovenous pressure gradient is subnormal. However, this inherent compensatory mechanism is soon overcome by a developing ACS whereby venous blood flow is inhibited by the raised intramuscular pressure, thus lowering the arteriovenous gradient.
2. Another compensatory coping strategy utilised by ischaemic muscle is to extract more oxygen than is the norm from venous blood. In non-ischaemic situations, oxygen delivery is excessive; and therefore, the venous blood contains surplus oxygen that can be utilised when the body is exercising and the demand for oxygen is higher. A decline in pH will favour an increase in oxygen offloading due to a shift in the haemoglobin dissociation curve, and in the presence of a developing ACS, this mechanism for obtaining additional oxygen is maximised.
3. The third and most important coping mechanism is the ability of all human cells to generate energy in the presence of ischaemia by activating the glycolytic pathway. Although the mechanism is effective, it is not an efficient use of glucose since it results in 12-fold lower production of ATP compared with oxidative phosphorylation and produces lactic acid as a by-product. Glycolysis is employed by all cells on a routine basis and is activated when required to make up any energy shortfall. In the presence of a developing ACS, the glycolytic pathway becomes increasingly important for cell survival, although, through its inefficiencies, it is not sustainable, and ATP production declines to a level where adequate plasma and organelle membrane function is lost, and reversible cell injury becomes irreversible.

Could biochemical markers be indicative of impending irreversible cell injury?

In principle, if the tissue concentrations of key biochemical markers could be measured accurately, it seems likely that a relationship between their concentration and the extent of tissue ischaemia could be established. However, these potential relationships have not been investigated in depth, and to date no studies have been undertaken that directly compare the biochemical composition of muscle with the morphological features of reversible and irreversible cell injury.

Through research undertaken in our unit, we have investigated the potential relationship between progressive ischaemia in skeletal muscle with the tissue concentration of key biomarker molecules (glucose-6-phosphate, pyruvate and lactate) that play central roles in oxidative phosphorylation and glycolysis, and the end products, ATP. The model that we used was a non-circulatory model utilising fresh avascular blocks of mammal skeletal muscle. Although this model is not directly comparable with ACS models, where the blood flow is gradually deteriorating, our model was useful due to its simplicity, consistency and ability to foreshorten the overall experimental time from well-vascularised muscle to irreversible cell injury (death). The experimental model also facilitated the process of obtaining biopsy specimens at regular intervals. After freezing all biopsy specimens in liquid nitrogen and further processing of the specimens, we were able to measure the tissue concentration of each of the aforementioned key molecules and compare them in relation to ischaemic duration and level of tissue pH with the latter being calculated using the aerobic–anaerobic equation described by Sahlin [10] and used to determine the extent of ischaemia. The aerobic–anaerobic equation is dependent upon the concentrations of lactate and pyruvate, which are key intermediate and end molecules in the glycolytic and oxidative pathways. They are therefore indicative of the balance between anaerobic and aerobic respiration. Tissue concentrations of ATP and PCr were used to determine when the cell energy reserves were depleted to the point of irreversible cell injury and cell death was imminent.

In summary, over time, glucose-6-phosphate, pyruvate levels and PCr decline predictably as these key energy substrates are used to make ATP (Figs. 4.1, 4.2, and 4.3). In response to the glycolytic activity, lactate levels increase over time (Fig. 4.4). Finally, despite the concerted effort to maintain ATP re-synthesis, the metabolic consequence of ischaemia still results in a ~75% decline ATP concentration after 90 minutes (Fig. 4.5).

In addition, when the tissue concentrations of all of these molecules are plotted against tissue pH (data not shown), there is a strong correlation (and a reverse correlation for lactate) between both pH and the concentrations of the aforementioned key molecules.

Assuming that there is a relationship between the concentration of key biochemical markers and the extent of muscle ischaemia, could any of these markers be used as an objective measure of ischaemia?

Our research strongly suggests that a number of these biochemical markers could be useful in determining the extent of tissue ischaemia, irrespective of the cause, but the difficulty lies in how best to measure their concentration in tissues in the clinical setting. Microdialysis is one method that could be employed, but this technique which can be used to measure the extracellular concentration of molecules of interest would be questionable under conditions when an increase in the intramuscular pressure may

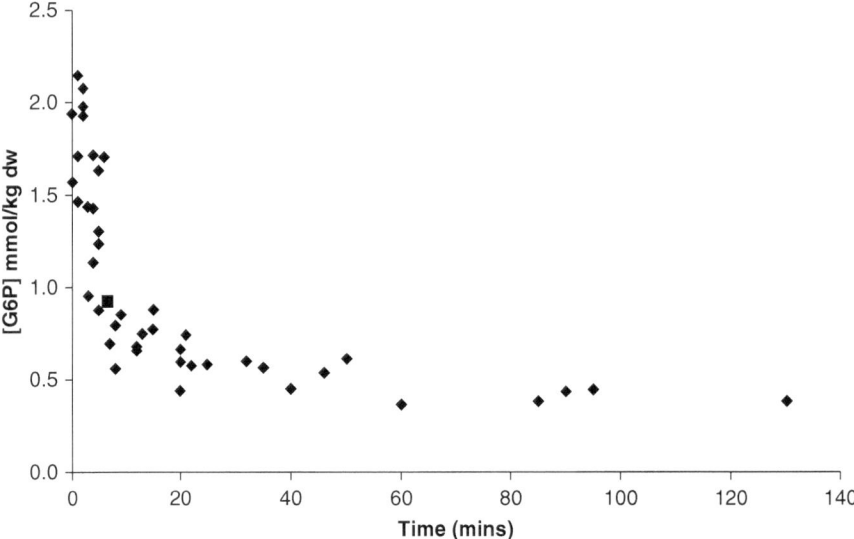

Fig. 4.1 Ischaemic mammalian animal muscle study: glucose-6-phosphate concentration against time

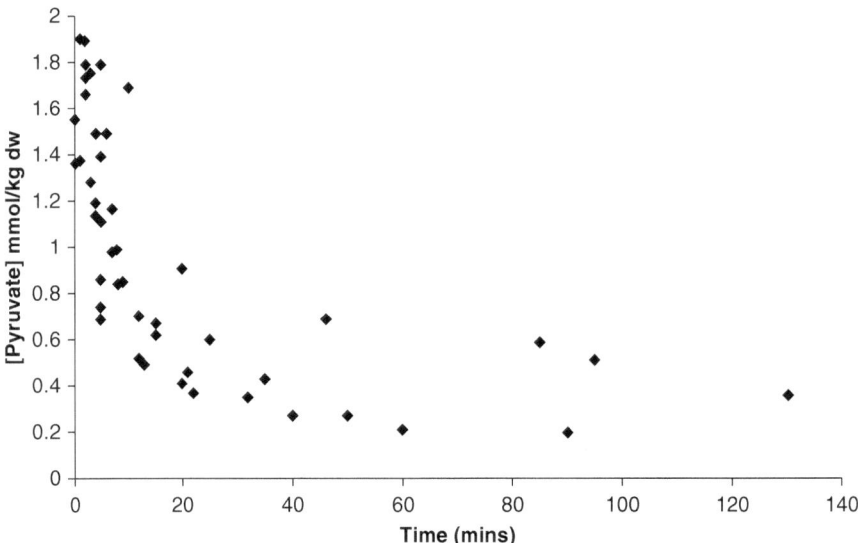

Fig. 4.2 Ischaemic mammalian animal muscle study: pyruvate concentration against time

influence the movement of biomolecular markers in contrast to normal conditions. In principle, spectrophotometric methods for determining the tissue concentration of these key molecules hold promise but would require multi-wavelength optical analysis for each metabolite of interest and as such are not sufficiently well advanced to be

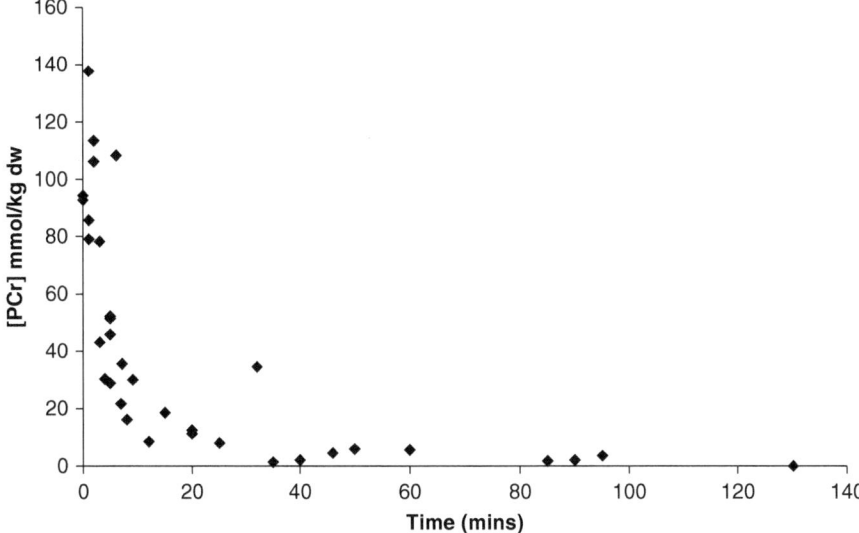

Fig. 4.3 Ischaemic mammalian animal muscle study: phosphocreatine concentration against time

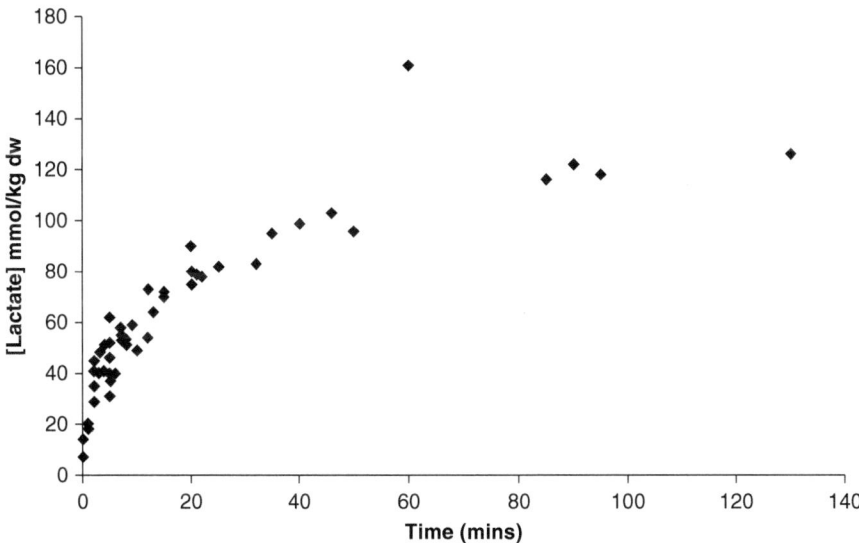

Fig. 4.4 Ischaemic mammalian animal muscle study: lactate concentration against time

of use. Even the more established spectrophotometric technique for determining the oxygen concentration in tissues, near-infrared spectroscopy (NIRS) is not proving to be as useful as was first anticipated due to a number of confounding factors.

One method that we have been investigating in more detail is the potential of measuring pH directly in muscle. Tissue acidity (pH) is a direct reflection of the

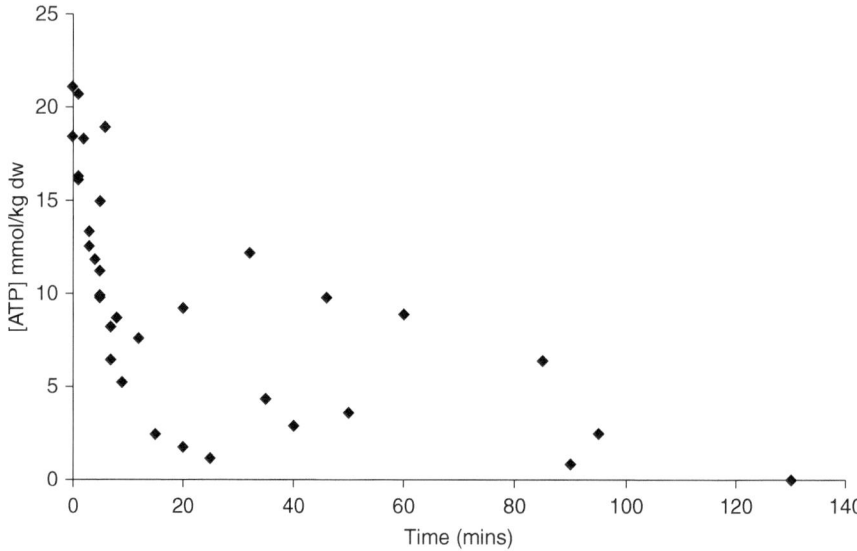

Fig. 4.5 Ischaemic mammalian animal muscle study: ATP concentration against time

concentration of H^+ ions present, and although the H^+ ion is not one of the key molecules, it does represent a reasonably accurate measure of glycolysis that has been taking place. In addition to the aforementioned biochemical analyses, our experiments also assessed the accuracy of measuring directly the tissue pH of muscle using pH probes. Our results confirmed a strong correlation ($R^2 = 0.926$) between directly measured pH with calculated pH based upon the tissue concentration of lactate and pyruvate, using the aerobic–anaerobic equation. Although more work is required to confirm the earlier findings, it is possible that directly measured tissue acidity using a pH probe may prove to be a useful objective measure of muscular metabolic status related to ischaemia that could have roles in diagnosing and assessing the severity of ACS in addition to other forms of compartment syndrome [11].

Limitations of Current Knowledge and Future Directions

- It is clear that further research needs to be done in an attempt to directly associate the concentrations of key cellular metabolic markers with the morphological changes that are recognised for reversible and irreversible cell injury. If key metabolic biomarkers can be identified, these will open the door to the development of new objective measures of ischaemia.
- Based on our research (laboratory and clinical), monitoring intramuscular pH seems to be a highly accurate method (high sensitivity and specificity) for detecting muscle ischaemia and the metabolic status of the muscle and appears to have

advantages over ICP monitoring. A future RCT will be required to assess the potential of IMpH monitoring to diagnose ACS and other forms of compartment syndrome [12].

Take-Home Message
- Skeletal muscle is a highly metabolically active tissue that has a constant demand for energy.
- Underlying cellular metabolic pathways are well established for both aerobic and anaerobic environments.
- Morphological changes in cellular structure have also been well described for both reversible and irreversible cell damage secondary to ischaemia.
- Identifying key stages in the cellular metabolic response to ischaemia that can differentiate between reversible and irreversible cell damage (ischaemic threshold) should be possible.
- Identifying an ischaemic threshold is of fundamental importance if new diagnostic methods are to be developed that would aid the decision-making process of clinicians responsible for treating patients with a suspected compartment syndrome or other forms of peripheral ischaemia.
- Early research suggests that direct intramuscular pH monitoring could be a suitable objective measure of muscle ischaemia including compartment syndrome.
- Despite enthusiastic attempts to diagnose peripheral ischaemia by measuring key biochemical markers in venous or arterial blood, dilutional effects significantly dampen the responsiveness of potential markers except in extreme situations where extensive ischaemic damage resulting in cell death is present, by which time, treatment is aimed at tissue/limb salvage at best.

References

1. Elliott KGB, Johnstone AJ. Diagnosing acute compartment syndrome. Bone Joint J. 2003;85-B:625–32.
2. Williams PR, Russell D, Mintowt-Cryz WJ. Compartment pressure monitoring – current UK orthopaedic practice. Injury. 1998;29:229–32.
3. Wall CJ, Richardson MD, Lowe AJ, Brand C, Lynch J, de Steiger RN. Survey of management of acute traumatic compartment syndrome of the leg in Australia. ANZ J Surg. 2007;9:733–7.
4. Smith IC, Bombardier E, Vigna C, Tupling AR. ATP consumption by sarcoplasmic reticulum Ca2+ pumps accounts for 40-50% of resting metabolic rate in mouse fast and slow twitch skeletal muscle. PlosOne. 2013;8(7):e68924. PMID: 23840903.
5. Hultman E, Spriet LL. Skeletal muscle metabolism, contraction force and glycogen utilization during prolonged electrical stimulation in humans. J Physiol. 1986;374:493–501. Hultman E, Sjoholm H. Energy metabolism and contraction force of human skeletal muscle in situ during electrical stimulation. J Physiol. 1983;345:525–32.

6. Jones N. Hydrogen ion balance during exercise. Clin Sci. 1980;59:85–91.
7. Wahren J, Felig P, Ahlborg G, Jorfeldt L. Glucose metabolism during exercise in man. J Clin Invest. 1972;50:2715–25.
8. Ball D. Metabolic and endocrine response to exercise: sympathoadrenal integration with skeletal muscle. J Endocrinol. 2015;224:R79-95; Meyer RA, Terjung RL. AMP deamination and IMP reamination in working skeletal muscle. Am J Phys. 1980;239:C32–8.
9. Patton MS. A review of the underlying biochemistry of muscle ischaemia in relation to intramuscular pH measurements. MD Thesis, University of Aberdeen, 2008. (unpublished).
10. Sahlin K. Muscle energetics during explosive activities and potential effects of nutrition and training. Sports Med. 2014;44:S167–73.
11. Elliott KGB. Intramuscular pH as a novel diagnostic tool for acute compartment syndrome: a prospective clinical study. MD Thesis, University of Aberdeen, 2007.
12. Schmidt AH, Bosse MJ, Frey KP, O'Toole RV, Stinner DJ, Scharfstein DO, Zipunnikov V, MacKenzie EJ, METRC. Predicting acute compartment syndrome (PACS): the role of continuous monitoring. J Orthop Trauma. 2017;31(Suppl 1):S40–7.

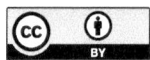

Chapter 5
Pressure Measurement: Surrogate of Ischaemia

Andrew D. Duckworth, Charles M. Court-Brown, and Margaret M. McQueen

Background to the Problem

- It is well established that the expedient diagnosis of acute compartment syndrome (ACS), followed by urgent fasciotomy and decompression, provides the best outcome for the patient by avoiding irreversible tissue ischaemia and necrosis [1–4].
- Delay in the diagnosis of ACS can lead to potentially catastrophic outcomes for the patient [5–9], as well as being associated with high medical costs [10] and medicolegal indemnity cases [11, 12]. Complications include infection, muscle necrosis/contractures, nerve injury, chronic pain, fracture non-union and even amputation.
- Factors associated with a delay/failure of diagnosis are inadequate experience of medical personnel, regional or general anaesthesia (GA), polytrauma patients, soft tissue injuries as well as the use of clinical signs alone when making the diagnosis [4, 13–20].
- There is currently no universally agreed reference standard for the diagnosis of ACS, and the prevalence documented in literature is below 30%, meaning the diagnostic performance characteristics of any test is by definition limited [21–23].
- The use of intra-compartmental pressure (ICP) monitoring continues to be debated, with one study using it as the primary diagnostic tool in only 11.7% of 386 tibial shaft fractures [23], whilst a recent survey of US trauma surgeons

A. D. Duckworth (✉)
Edinburgh Orthopedic Trauma Unit, Royal Infirmary of Edinburgh, Edinburgh, UK
e-mail: andrew.duckworth@ed.ac.uk

C. M. Court-Brown · M. M. McQueen
University of Edinburgh, Edinburgh, UK

© The Author(s) 2019
C. Mauffrey et al. (eds.), *Compartment Syndrome*,
https://doi.org/10.1007/978-3-030-22331-1_5

reported that clinical assessment should be utilised in the awake patient, with monitoring recommended in the obtunded or unconscious patient [24]

What Is Recommended?

Which Patients Should Be Monitored?

The incidence of acute compartment syndrome (ACS) is documented to be 3.1 per 100,000 population/year [21]. Males are more frequently affected than females (10:1) [21, 25], and the mean age is quoted at just over 30 years, with males younger than females [21, 26, 27]. Table 5.1 details those patients in whom compartment pressure monitoring is recommended. These can be considered risk factors and/or high-risk patients for the development of ACS, as well as factors known to be associated with a delayed diagnosis of ACS [4, 13–20].

Youth is the principal risk factor for developing ACS, with the highest prevalence documented to be in the second and third decades [29]. One proposed explanation for this is that young patients have a higher muscle bulk and thus a limited capacity for swelling in a fixed compartment. Sarcopenia and an associated increased perfusion pressure due to hypertension can also possibly explain the protective effects of ageing. The important caveat for youth as a risk factor are cases of ACS secondary to soft tissue injuries, which make up almost a quarter of all cases [1, 30, 31]. For these cases, it is noted that the mean age is significantly older than those who develop ACS following a fracture [32]. Soft tissue causes of ACS include crush injuries, crush syndrome, drug overdose and anticoagulant medications [16, 21, 27, 33–40].

Table 5.1 Patients at high risk of ACS and where pressure monitoring is recommended

Patients in who pressure monitoring is recommended
Youth
Tibial fractures
High-energy forearm fractures
High-energy femoral diaphyseal fractures
Patients with a background of bleeding disorders and/or anticoagulants
Polytrauma patients
High base deficit
High lactate levels
Transfusion requirement
Altered conscious level
Regional anaesthesia or patient-controlled analgesia
Children and/or adolescents with at-risk injuries
Patients with associated nerve injuries
Table adapted from Duckworth and McQueen [28]

Tibial diaphyseal fractures account for a third of all ACS cases [21]. Despite some previous literature suggesting that intramedullary nailing was associated with the development of ACS [7, 41–45], other studies have found this not to be the case [45, 46], and more recently, youth, males and diaphyseal fractures are noted to be the key risk factors [4, 22]. Recent literature has reported an increased risk of ACS following tibial plateau fractures [47], particularly the more complex higher-energy Schatzker VI types [47, 48]. Forearm diaphyseal fractures and fractures of the distal radius, particularly high-energy, are also associated with ACS.

The current literature suggests a high rate of ACS following closed low-energy rather than open high-energy fractures of the tibial shaft [21, 49–51]. The reason for this could be due to the theory of 'auto-decompression' of the fascial boundaries at the time of injury. However, there is data to certainly support an increased rate of ACS following high-energy forearm and femoral fractures [21, 25, 38, 52]. One study has reported a lower limb ACS rate of 20% in critically injured patients, with increased lactate levels and base deficit, as well as a transfusion need associated with the diagnosis [53].

What Are the Techniques Available?

The advantages and disadvantages of the various invasive monitoring techniques available are found in Table 5.2. The needle manometer [54–56] was an early method of pressure monitoring and is a simple and cheap technique, but there are noted problems with the tip blocking and major concerns associated with the large volume of fluid infused, which could induce or exacerbate compartment syndrome. The wick catheter was a modification of this [57, 58] and provides a large surface area for pressure measurement, whilst also reducing the blocking risk. However, false low measurements have been noted if a blockage (e.g. blood clot or air bubble) does occur.

The slit catheter is like the wick catheter [59–61] and is the technique we use in our centre [62]. Again, a large surface area is available for measurement via an axial cut at the catheter end [59]. Patency can be assessed when the catheter is in place by applying light pressure to the compartment, which should give an immediate transient elevation in the pressure reading. The data suggests that the slit catheter is superior to the needle manometer method [60] and comparable to the wick catheter [61].

A solid-state transducer intra-compartmental catheter (STIC) can also be used to measure compartment pressures [63–65]. This method employs a pressure transducer within the catheter lumen. Good correlations with conventional techniques have been reported [64]; however, this method is expensive/labour intensive, and less modern designs can require an infusion to maintain patency [65]. There is also the Stryker ICP™ monitor (Stryker, Kalamazoo, MI), which is commonly used in North America for compartment pressure monitoring. The accuracy of this monitor has been shown to be limited as regards inter-observer variability [66].

Table 5.2 The advantages and disadvantages of the currently available ICP monitoring techniques used in the diagnosis of acute compartment syndrome

Method	Advantages	Disadvantages
Needle manometer	Simple technique Low cost	Accuracy limited with false positives/negatives Invasive indirect measure Continuous measurement unfeasible Needle tip may block Fluid infusion can cause clinical picture to deteriorate
Wick catheter	Good accuracy with high surface area Blockage of catheter uncommon Continuous monitoring feasible	Invasive indirect measure Blockage at air/fluid junction possible Wick material retention possible Transducer must be at catheter level
Transducer-tip intra-compartmental catheter	Good accuracy Continuous monitoring feasible Transducer level not important	Increased costs Re-sterilisation necessary
Slit catheter	Good accuracy with high surface area Continuous monitoring feasible	Invasive indirect measure Catheter may block Air bubble can lead to false low reading Transducer must be at catheter level
Near-infrared spectroscopy	Good accuracy and correlation Continuous monitoring feasible Non-invasive technique	Increased costs Not yet clearly validated for ACS Measurement dependant on soft tissue depth

Reproduced from Duckworth and McQueen [28]

Where Should the Catheter Be Placed?

The recommended catheter placement location for the upper and lower limb sites at risk of ACS is found in Table 5.3. Accurate catheter placement within the affected compartment is carried out using a strict aseptic technique [67]. In the presence of a fracture, the literature would suggest that the catheter tip should be placed within 5 cm of the level of the fracture, as this will give the peak measure reading within the compartment [4, 68–70]. Others advocate this results in a false high reading due to the fracture haematoma [71]. It is essential that the transducer is secured at the level of the compartment as the readings will to change with the height relative to the compartment.

Current data would suggest the lower leg anterior compartment should be used as it is the most commonly involved compartment and is easily accessible [51, 72]. However, some authors advocate concomitant monitoring of the deep posterior

Table 5.3 The recommended catheter placement location for the upper and lower limb sites at risk of ACS

Location	Recommended location for catheter placement
Upper limb	
Arm	Anterior compartment (posterior if clinically suspected)
Forearm	Flexor/volar compartment (extensor/dorsal if clinically suspected)
Hand	Interosseous compartments
Lower limb	
Thigh	Anterior compartment
Lower leg	Anterior compartment (deep posterior if clinically suspected)
Foot	Interosseous compartments (calcaneal compartment for hindfoot injuries)

compartment due to the possibility of missing an isolated deep ACS. It should be noted that this is often uncomfortable and cumbersome for the patient [5, 68].

What Is the Pressure Threshold for Decompression?

There has been much debate when using compartment pressure monitoring regarding the pressure threshold for diagnosing ACS and proceeding to fasciotomy. Should we use the absolute compartment pressure in isolation? Is the differential pressure or perfusion pressure (ΔP) the best thing to use?

Early data suggested using an absolute ICP threshold of 30–40 mmHg [30, 50, 54, 58, 73–75]. However, it was subsequently noted that a patient's tolerance for an absolute pressure reading does vary widely and was intrinsically linked with the systemic blood pressure or perfusion pressure [51, 69, 76–78]. Whitesides et al. documented the use of the differential pressure (ΔP), calculated as diastolic pressure − intra-compartmental pressure [76]. Following on from this, data then proposed a differential pressure of 10–35 mmHg as diagnostic [69, 78, 79]. However, it has been noted that the differential pressure will possibly be increased in traumatised or ischaemic muscle.

There is now clinical and experimental data supporting a differential pressure of ≤ 30 mmHg as diagnostic for ACS requiring fasciotomy [6, 51, 67, 80]. In a study from our centre, there were 116 patients with an acute fracture of the tibial shaft [51] that underwent immediate continuous pressure monitoring of the anterior compartment for a minimum of 24 hours. The authors used a differential pressure of ≤ 30 mmHg for more than 2 hours as diagnostic, with 3 patients requiring fasciotomy. No unnecessary fasciotomies were noted, and there were no missed cases of ACS and no related sequelae at a final mean follow-up of just over a year [51].

This protocol was subsequently validated in our centre by White et al. in a study of 101 tibial diaphyseal fractures. In this series, 41 patients had an absolute pressure reading of greater than 30 mmHg for more than 6 hours continuously, but with a normal differential pressure of >30 mmHg. These patients were compared with 60 patients who all had an absolute reading of less than 30 mmHg throughout. In the year following intervention, no significant difference in isometric muscle analysis or in return to function was found between these two groups [67].

Janzing et al. assessed a monitoring protocol in a prospective study of 95 patients with a tibial shaft fracture that underwent continuous pressure monitoring [81]. There was a 14.4% fasciotomy rate reported in the series. The authors found that the optimal combined sensitivity and specificity was clinical symptoms *and* differential pressure of <30 mmHg (61%, 97%), with a differential pressure of ≤30 mmHg performing best when using monitoring alone (89%, 65%). The authors suggested that an increased fasciotomy rate could occur with continuous pressure monitoring, but this study does not completely consider the trend of the differential pressure over time.

Is Continuous Monitoring Important?

Time to fasciotomy is established to be a key factor in predicting patient outcome [5–9]. All the available data clearly determines that timing is of critical importance in the development of muscle damage [73, 75, 82, 83]. However, it is also necessary to contemplate the trend over time for compartment pressure monitoring in order to confirm the diagnosis of ACS and determine the need to proceed to fasciotomy, with the exception of severe or extreme cases that obviously need to proceed to theatre immediately. The current data suggests that if a single pressure reading is used, then this will most probably result in an increased rate of unnecessary fasciotomies (overtreatment). One study reported a false-positive rate of 35% if a one-off differential pressure reading of ≤30 mmHg was used as diagnostic and if the trend over time was not considered [84].

Kakar et al. reported a prospective study of 242 tibial shaft fractures treated with intramedullary nailing under general anaesthesia (GA) [85]. They found that although the preoperative diastolic blood pressure was related to the post-operative pressure, a significant difference was found with the intraoperative pressure. This work emphasises the need to use serial continuous measurements and that intraoperative and immediate post-operative readings should be used with caution. This is certainly the experience in our centre too.

The protocol we use in our centre is well documented in the literature, and when employing a differential pressure of ≤30 mmHg over a 2 hour period as diagnostic [62], we have reported a reduction in the time to fasciotomy and complication rate, whilst not significantly increasing the rate of fasciotomies [51]. We would suggest that if the differential pressure is below 30 mmHg, but the absolute pressure is decreasing (and thus the differential pressure is increasing), then it is most likely safe to closely observe the patient in the expectation of the differential pressure returning to safe levels within a short period of time.

How Do Clinical Signs Compare with Pressure Monitoring?

To determine whether pressure measurement is a good surrogate for ischaemia, it is important to consider what the alternatives are, namely, clinical assessment. The clinical symptoms and signs associated with the development of ACS are swelling, pain on passive stretch, pain out of proportion to the injury, paraesthesia and paresis/paralysis. The diagnostic performance characteristics of these symptoms and signs are found in Table 5.4.

Swelling is almost a universally seen sign with all the causes of ACS and is very subjective. Despite pain being an important early symptom of ACS in the awake and alert patient [15], it is common after most injuries, is very subjective/patient dependent and is not universally present in all cases of ACS [88]. Pain assessment is also not possible when regional anaesthesia has been used or in the unconscious patient [13, 14, 18]. Pain has a low sensitivity and a large false-negative/missed cases rate reported in the literature [5, 6, 15, 33, 89]. Paraesthesia or reduced sensation is now established as a late sign of ACS [8] with a very low sensitivity and a rate of false negatives [15]. This rate of false negatives excludes paraesthesia as an accurate diagnostic indicator. Paralysis of the muscles within compartment is also a very late sign of ACS and is indicative of irreversible damage to the soft tissues within the compartment. It is associated with a poor outcome [30, 31, 38, 49, 90, 91] and has the worst combined sensitivity and specificity in the literature [15]. Vascular assessment is not an early clinical sign of ACS, with absent peripheral pulses, pallor and reduced capillary refill time all associated with either an acute vascular injury that needs an urgent angiogram/intervention or possibly an established ACS where an amputation is very possible [4]. Importantly, it is also not possible to rule out ACS due to strong distal pulses.

Some studies have tried to directly compare the use of clinical assessment alone with compartment pressure monitoring. In a study from our centre, we reported on 25 patients with a tibial shaft fracture that developed ACS [6]. There were 13 patients who underwent compartment pressure monitoring and 12 patients who had clinical assessment alone. There was a significant delayed time from presentation to fasciotomy for the non-monitored group (16 hour difference;

Table 5.4 The reported sensitivities and specificities of the clinical symptoms and signs of ACS, along with the diagnostic performance characteristics of ICP monitoring

Symptom or sign	Sensitivity (%)	Specificity (%)	PPV (%)	NPV (%)
Pain [15]	19	97	14	98
Pain on passive stretch [15]	19	97	14	98
Paresis/motor changes [15]	13	97	11	98
Paraesthesia/sensory changes [15]	13	98	15	98
Swelling [86]	54	76	70	63
ICP monitoring [87]	94	98	93	99

Reproduced from Duckworth and McQueen [28]
PPV positive predictive value, *NPV* negative predictive value, *ICP* intra-compartmental pressure

$p < 0.05$), with also a significantly increased rate of late sequelae (91% vs. 0%; $p < 0.01$) and delay to union (8 week delay; $p < 0.05$) [6].

A further study reported on 218 patients that included 109 consecutive tibial shaft fractures that had continuous compartment pressure monitoring and retrospectively compared them with 109 control patients that underwent clinical assessment only [72]. The authors reported comparable rates of fasciotomy (15.6% vs. 14.7%). However, there was no significant difference in either patient outcome or time to fasciotomy [72]. One potential criticism of this study is that the control group had clinical examination performed hourly, which could be argued to be inconsistent with routine clinical practice.

Harris et al. are the only authors, to our knowledge, to have carried out a prospective randomised trial [71]. Their study included 200 consecutive tibial shaft fractures and randomised patients to clinical assessment alone ($n = 100$) or compartment pressure monitoring ($n = 100$). All five cases of ACS in the study were in the clinical assessment group. The authors chose a primary outcome of late ACS sequelae at the six-month assessment. Complications that were reported included sensory loss, muscle weakness, contractures and toe clawing, and fracture non-union. There was no significant difference in overall complication rates found between groups (27% vs. 29%). A potential criticism of this study was that the indication for fasciotomy was clinical assessment, with monitoring only employed at the discretion of the treating surgeon [71].

Diagnostic Performance Characteristics (Table 5.4)

The diagnostic performance characteristics of continuous invasive compartment pressure monitoring and those of clinical symptoms/signs are found in Table 5.4. Our centre has reported on a series of 850 adult patients with an acute tibial shaft fracture using a slit catheter technique in the anterior compartment of the leg and a diagnostic pressure threshold differential (ΔP) of less than 30 mmHg for more than 2 hours as indication for fasciotomy [87]. We reported high diagnostic performance characteristics, with 11 false-positive cases and 9 false-negative cases. In order to attain comparable characteristics to these, Ulmer et al. found in their systematic review of clinical assessment that three clinical signs are needed, with the third being paralysis – a sign associated with irreversible damage to the muscle [15]. Symptoms and signs in isolation were also found to perform poorly and are known to be better at ruling out rather than confirming the diagnosis (Table 5.4).

Limitations and Pitfalls

ACS continues to be a catastrophic complication and is associated with significant patient morbidity and high litigation costs [11, 92]. A review from Canada over a 10-year period reported that 77% of plaintiffs had permanent disability and 55% of cases had a judgement for the plaintiff or an unfavourable decision for the physician, with the primary clinical issue a delay or failure to diagnose ACS [92]. Despite all this evidence highlighting the issues with a delay in the diagnosis, there remains an extraordinary lack of consistency in the clinical assessment of the condition [93, 94].

A key limitation of the literature on ACS is how we define the time of onset of acute compartment syndrome (e.g. when the diagnosis was made), as well as the time to fasciotomy. In the acute trauma clinical setting, authors have suggested that the time to fasciotomy is best determined as the point from admission as this is the most likely easily definable moment in the patient journey [4, 32, 51]. The obvious exception to this is crush syndrome, as the nature of the diagnosis is associated with a prolonged period of compression that makes it almost impossible to determine the exact time of onset.

The current data is also deficient in good quality prospective mid-term and long-term outcome data on the efficacy of compartment pressure monitoring, as well as the outcome of fasciotomy and ACS. There is also very little literature reporting on the various diagnostic performance characteristics for the pressure measurement techniques available, nor for the diagnostic protocols associated with these. Much of the data in the literature relates to adults and the lower leg. More data is needed on ACS in adolescent patients, as well as for other areas of the body. This would potentially then allow us to establish the indications, thresholds and protocols for using pressure monitoring in these patient groups. In children, given the normally lower diastolic pressure in this patient group, the mean arterial pressure (MAP) might be a preferred option when calculating the differential pressure [95].

Finally, one of the key problems with the current literature on the diagnosis of ACS is the absence of an agreed gold-standard reference. Given the incidence is known to be below 30% [21–23], routine statistical methods are not likely rigorous enough. Alternative methods such as latent class analysis and Bayes theorem are required to accurately calculate the diagnostic performance characteristics of the various methods used.

Future Directions

Given the superior published diagnostic performance characteristics of continuous pressure monitoring when compared to clinical symptoms and signs, a clinical diagnosis alone of ACS we feel should not be the gold standard. Continuous pressure monitoring is of benefit in all patients at risk of developing ACS, and universally clear and accepted clinical guidelines are needed to allow the early diagnosis in all units managing acute trauma patients. This would, most probably, result in the single biggest advance in the management of the condition. Clearly, the ultimate goal would be a sufficiently powered large multicentre prospective randomised controlled trial of the clinical signs of ACS versus continuous pressure monitoring. However, the 'Hawthorn effect' comes into play here due to the probability of modifying what is normal day-to-day clinical practice, due to the predictable improvement in the frequency and rigour of the clinical assessment for such a trial.

The role of non-invasive compartment pressure measurements and those measuring blood flow continue to be investigated in the literature [96]. The potential advantages are without question, but the utilisation of these techniques is thus far not been sufficiently validated in the literature. Near-infrared spectroscopy utilises a probe placed on the skin to determine the degree of oxygenated haemoglobin in the muscle tissues [97–100]. It has been shown to correlate well with tissue pressures from experimental data [97], as well as in healthy human volunteers [98]. The role of ultrasound scanning to detect waveforms associated with displacement of the fascia by the arterial pulse continues to be unclear. There has been investigations trying to correlate compartment pressure readings of greater than 30 mmHg with fascial displacement in healthy volunteers, with the reported sensitivity 77% and specificity 93% [101]. The clear limitation of this technique is the likely reduction in sensitivity for the hypotensive patient.

Methods to prevent or reduce the effects of ACS are also potential areas for future work. Research has already started on methods to reduce the compartment pressure with the administration of intravenously hypertonic fluids [102], but these have never been successful clinically. Nevertheless, an experiment on human subjects using tissue ultrafiltration to remove fluid from the compartment has been shown to reduce compartment pressure [103, 104]. Whether this technique can be useful clinically remains to be seen. There is also work on the potential role of antioxidants on the outcome of ACS with some promising findings reported [105], with extension into human studies the next step.

Take-Home Message

- Pain is documented as the index sign associated with the development of acute compartment syndrome. However, clinical symptoms and signs in isolation are reported to have inadequate diagnostic performance characteristics, with the sensitivity ranging from 13% to 54% for each in the literature.
- Continuous invasive intra-compartmental pressure monitoring has been reported to have superior diagnostic performance characteristics with a high estimated sensitivity (94%) and specificity (98%) for the diagnosis of ACS when using a slit catheter technique and a differential pressure threshold of 30 mmHg for more than 2 hours.
- Continuous pressure monitoring should be utilised as a diagnostic adjunct in all patients at risk of developing ACS, with youth the key risk factor and tibial diaphyseal fractures the most common precipitating injury identified in the literature.
- Patients and surgeons need to acknowledge that when using compartment pressure monitoring for diagnosing ACS, the risk should inevitably lean towards an unnecessary fasciotomy (false positive) rather than a missed ACS (false negative).
- Future non-invasive techniques of calculating tissue perfusion via blood flow or pH remain areas of future research, along with interventions that can potentially reduce the effects of ACS.

References

1. Gelberman RH, Zakaib GS, Mubarak SJ, Hargens AR, Akeson WH. Decompression of forearm compartment syndromes. Clin Orthop Relat Res. 1978;134:225–9.
2. Holden CE. The pathology and prevention of Volkmann's ischaemic contracture. J Bone Joint Surg Br. 1979;61-B(3):296–300.
3. Finkelstein JA, Hunter GA, Hu RW. Lower limb compartment syndrome: course after delayed fasciotomy. J Trauma. 1996;40(3):342–4.
4. McQueen MM. Acute compartment syndrome. In: Bucholz RW, Court-Brown CM, Heckman JD, Tornetta III P, editors. Rockwood and Green's fractures in adults. 7th ed. Philadelphia: Lippincott Williams & Wilkins; 2010. p. 689–708.
5. Matsen FA III, Clawson DK. The deep posterior compartmental syndrome of the leg. J Bone Joint Surg Am. 1975;57(1):34–9.
6. McQueen MM, Christie J, Court-Brown CM. Acute compartment syndrome in tibial diaphyseal fractures. J Bone Joint Surg Br. 1996;78(1):95–8.
7. Mullett H, Al-Abed K, Prasad CV, O'Sullivan M. Outcome of compartment syndrome following intramedullary nailing of tibial diaphyseal fractures. Injury. 2001;32(5):411–3.
8. Rorabeck CH, Macnab L. Anterior tibial-compartment syndrome complicating fractures of the shaft of the tibia. J Bone Joint Surg Am. 1976;58(4):549–50.
9. Sheridan GW, Matsen FA III. Fasciotomy in the treatment of the acute compartment syndrome. J Bone Joint Surg Am. 1976;58(1):112–5.
10. Schmidt AH. The impact of compartment syndrome on hospital length of stay and charges among adult patients admitted with a fracture of the tibia. J Orthop Trauma. 2011;25(6): 355–7.
11. Bhattacharyya T, Vrahas MS. The medical-legal aspects of compartment syndrome. J Bone Joint Surg Am. 2004;86-A(4):864–8.
12. Matsen FA III, Stephens L, Jette JL, Warme WJ, Posner KL. Lessons regarding the safety of orthopaedic patient care: an analysis of four hundred and sixty-four closed malpractice claims. J Bone Joint Surg Am. 2013;95(4):e201–8.
13. Mubarak SJ, Wilton NC. Compartment syndromes and epidural analgesia. J Pediatr Orthop. 1997;17(3):282–4.
14. Harrington P, Bunola J, Jennings AJ, Bush DJ, Smith RM. Acute compartment syndrome masked by intravenous morphine from a patient-controlled analgesia pump. Injury. 2000;31(5):387–9.
15. Ulmer T. The clinical diagnosis of compartment syndrome of the lower leg: are clinical findings predictive of the disorder? J Orthop Trauma. 2002;16(8):572–7.
16. Mithofer K, Lhowe DW, Vrahas MS, Altman DT, Altman GT. Clinical spectrum of acute compartment syndrome of the thigh and its relation to associated injuries. Clin Orthop Relat Res. 2004;425:223–9.
17. Richards H, Langston A, Kulkarni R, Downes EM. Does patient controlled analgesia delay the diagnosis of compartment syndrome following intramedullary nailing of the tibia? Injury. 2004;35(3):296–8.
18. Davis ET, Harris A, Keene D, Porter K, Manji M. The use of regional anaesthesia in patients at risk of acute compartment syndrome. Injury. 2006;37(2):128–33.
19. Mar GJ, Barrington MJ, McGuirk BR. Acute compartment syndrome of the lower limb and the effect of postoperative analgesia on diagnosis. Br J Anaesth. 2009;102(1):3–11.
20. Roberts CS, Gorczyca JT, Ring D, Pugh KJ. Diagnosis and treatment of less common compartment syndromes of the upper and lower extremities: current evidence and best practices. Instr Course Lect. 2011;60:43–50.
21. McQueen MM, Gaston P, Court-Brown CM. Acute compartment syndrome. Who is at risk? J Bone Joint Surg Br. 2000;82(2):200–3.
22. Park S, Ahn J, Gee AO, Kuntz AF, Esterhai JL. Compartment syndrome in tibial fractures. J Orthop Trauma. 2009;23(7):514–8.

23. O'Toole RV, Whitney A, Merchant N, Hui E, Higgins J, Kim TT, et al. Variation in diagnosis of compartment syndrome by surgeons treating tibial shaft fractures. J Trauma. 2009;67(4):735–41.
24. Collinge CA, Attum B, Lebus GF, Tornetta P III, Obremskey W, Ahn J, et al. Acute compartment syndrome: an expert survey of orthopaedic trauma association members. J Orthop Trauma. 2018;32(5):e181–4.
25. Kalyani BS, Fisher BE, Roberts CS, Giannoudis PV. Compartment syndrome of the forearm: a systematic review. J Hand Surg Am. 2011;36(3):535–43.
26. Simpson NS, Jupiter JB. Delayed onset of forearm compartment syndrome: a complication of distal radius fracture in young adults. J Orthop Trauma. 1995;9(5):411–8.
27. Morin RJ, Swan KG, Tan V. Acute forearm compartment syndrome secondary to local arterial injury after penetrating trauma. J Trauma. 2009;66(4):989–93.
28. Duckworth AD, McQueen MM. The diagnosis of acute compartment syndrome: a critical analysis review. JBJS Rev. 2017;5(12):e1.
29. McQueen MM, Duckworth AD, Aitken SA, Sharma RA, Court-Brown CM. Predictors of compartment syndrome after Tibial fracture. J Orthop Trauma. 2015;29(10):451–5.
30. Rorabeck CH. The treatment of compartment syndromes of the leg. J Bone Joint Surg Br. 1984;66(1):93–7.
31. Bradley EL III. The anterior tibial compartment syndrome. Surg Gynecol Obstet. 1973;136(2):289–97.
32. Hope MJ, McQueen MM. Acute compartment syndrome in the absence of fracture. J Orthop Trauma. 2004;18(4):220–4.
33. Eaton RG, Green WT. Volkmann's ischemia. A volar compartment syndrome of the forearm. Clin Orthop Relat Res. 1975;113:58–64.
34. Mubarak S, Owen CA. Compartmental syndrome and its relation to the crush syndrome: a spectrum of disease. A review of 11 cases of prolonged limb compression. Clin Orthop Relat Res. 1975;113:81–9.
35. Reis ND, Michaelson M. Crush injury to the lower limbs. Treatment of the local injury. J Bone Joint Surg Am. 1986;68(3):414–8.
36. Gelberman RH, Garfin SR, Hergenroeder PT, Mubarak SJ, Menon J. Compartment syndromes of the forearm: diagnosis and treatment. Clin Orthop Relat Res. 1981;161:252–61.
37. Geary N. Late surgical decompression for compartment syndrome of the forearm. J Bone Joint Surg Br. 1984;66(5):745–8.
38. Schwartz JT Jr, Brumback RJ, Lakatos R, Poka A, Bathon GH, Burgess AR. Acute compartment syndrome of the thigh. A spectrum of injury. J Bone Joint Surg Am. 1989;71(3):392–400.
39. Mithofer K, Lhowe DW, Altman GT. Delayed presentation of acute compartment syndrome after contusion of the thigh. J Orthop Trauma. 2002;16(6):436–8.
40. Frink M, Hildebrand F, Krettek C, Brand J, Hankemeier S. Compartment syndrome of the lower leg and foot. Clin Orthop Relat Res. 2010;468(4):940–50.
41. Tischenko GJ, Goodman SB. Compartment syndrome after intramedullary nailing of the tibia. J Bone Joint Surg Am. 1990;72(1):41–4.
42. Moed BR, Strom DE. Compartment syndrome after closed intramedullary nailing of the tibia: a canine model and report of two cases. J Orthop Trauma. 1991;5(1):71–7.
43. Koval KJ, Clapper MF, Brumback RJ, Ellison PS Jr, Poka A, Bathon GH, et al. Complications of reamed intramedullary nailing of the tibia. J Orthop Trauma. 1991;5(2):184–9.
44. Williams J, Gibbons M, Trundle H, Murray D, Worlock P. Complications of nailing in closed tibial fractures. J Orthop Trauma. 1995;9(6):476–81.
45. Tornetta P III, French BG. Compartment pressures during nonreamed tibial nailing without traction. J Orthop Trauma. 1997;11(1):24–7.
46. McQueen MM, Christie J, Court-Brown CM. Compartment pressures after intramedullary nailing of the tibia. J Bone Joint Surg Br. 1990;72(3):395–7.
47. Allmon C, Greenwell P, Paryavi E, Dubina A, O'Toole RV. Radiographic predictors of compartment syndrome occurring after Tibial fracture. J Orthop Trauma. 2016;30(7):387–91.

48. Ziran BH, Becher SJ. Radiographic predictors of compartment syndrome in tibial plateau fractures. J Orthop Trauma. 2013;27(11):612–5.
49. DeLee JC, Stiehl JB. Open tibia fracture with compartment syndrome. Clin Orthop Relat Res. 1981;(160):175–84.
50. Blick SS, Brumback RJ, Poka A, Burgess AR, Ebraheim NA. Compartment syndrome in open tibial fractures. J Bone Joint Surg Am. 1986;68(9):1348–53.
51. McQueen MM, Court-Brown CM. Compartment monitoring in tibial fractures. The pressure threshold for decompression. J Bone Joint Surg Br. 1996;78(1):99–104.
52. Prasarn ML, Ouellette EA. Acute compartment syndrome of the upper extremity. J Am Acad Orthop Surg. 2011;19(1):49–58.
53. Kosir R, Moore FA, Selby JH, Cocanour CS, Kozar RA, Gonzalez EA, et al. Acute lower extremity compartment syndrome (ALECS) screening protocol in critically ill trauma patients. J Trauma. 2007;63(2):268–75.
54. Matsen FA III, Mayo KA, Sheridan GW, Krugmire RB Jr. Monitoring of intramuscular pressure. Surgery. 1976;79(6):702–9.
55. Matsen FA III, Winquist RA, Krugmire RB Jr. Diagnosis and management of compartmental syndromes. J Bone Joint Surg Am. 1980;62(2):286–91.
56. Whitesides TE Jr, Haney TC, Harada H, Holmes HE, Morimoto K. A simple method for tissue pressure determination. Arch Surg. 1975;110(11):1311–3.
57. Mubarak SJ, Hargens AR, Owen CA, Garetto LP, Akeson WH. The wick catheter technique for measurement of intramuscular pressure. A new research and clinical tool. J Bone Joint Surg Am. 1976;58(7):1016–20.
58. Mubarak SJ, Owen CA, Hargens AR, Garetto LP, Akeson WH. Acute compartment syndromes: diagnosis and treatment with the aid of the wick catheter. J Bone Joint Surg Am. 1978;60(8):1091–5.
59. Rorabeck CH, Castle GS, Hardie R, Logan J. Compartmental pressure measurements: an experimental investigation using the slit catheter. J Trauma. 1981;21(6):446–9.
60. Moed BR, Thorderson PK. Measurement of intracompartmental pressure: a comparison of the slit catheter, side-ported needle, and simple needle. J Bone Joint Surg Am. 1993;75(2):231–5.
61. Shakespeare DT, Henderson NJ, Clough G. The slit catheter: a comparison with the wick catheter in the measurement of compartment pressure. Injury. 1982;13(5):404–8.
62. Duckworth AD, McQueen MM. Continuous intracompartmental pressure monitoring for acute compartment syndrome. JBJS Essent Surg Tech. 2014;3(3):e13.
63. McDermott AG, Marble AE, Yabsley RH, Phillips MB. Monitoring dynamic anterior compartment pressures during exercise. A new technique using the STIC catheter. Am J Sports Med. 1982;10(2):83–9.
64. McDermott AG, Marble AE, Yabsley RH. Monitoring acute compartment pressures with the S.T.I.C. catheter. Clin Orthop Relat Res. 1984;190:192–8.
65. Willy C, Gerngross H, Sterk J. Measurement of intracompartmental pressure with use of a new electronic transducer-tipped catheter system. J Bone Joint Surg Am. 1999;81(2):158–68.
66. Large TM, Agel J, Holtzman DJ, Benirschke SK, Krieg JC. Interobserver variability in the measurement of lower leg compartment pressures. J Orthop Trauma. 2015;29(7):316–21.
67. White TO, Howell GE, Will EM, Court-Brown CM, McQueen MM. Elevated intramuscular compartment pressures do not influence outcome after tibial fracture. J Trauma. 2003;55(6):1133–8.
68. Heckman MM, Whitesides TE Jr, Grewe SR, Rooks MD. Compartment pressure in association with closed tibial fractures. The relationship between tissue pressure, compartment, and the distance from the site of the fracture. J Bone Joint Surg Am. 1994;76(9):1285–92.
69. Matava MJ, Whitesides TE Jr, Seiler JG III, Hewan-Lowe K, Hutton WC. Determination of the compartment pressure threshold of muscle ischemia in a canine model. J Trauma. 1994;37(1):50–8.
70. Saikia KC, Bhattacharya TD, Agarwala V. Anterior compartment pressure measurement in closed fractures of leg. Indian J Orthop. 2008;42(2):217–21.

71. Harris IA, Kadir A, Donald G. Continuous compartment pressure monitoring for tibia fractures: does it influence outcome? J Trauma. 2006;60(6):1330–5.
72. Al-Dadah OQ, Darrah C, Cooper A, Donell ST, Patel AD. Continuous compartment pressure monitoring vs. clinical monitoring in tibial diaphyseal fractures. Injury. 2008;39(10): 1204–9.
73. Hargens AR, Akeson WH, Mubarak SJ, Owen CA, Evans KL, Garetto LP, et al. Fluid balance within the canine anterolateral compartment and its relationship to compartment syndromes. J Bone Joint Surg Am. 1978;60(4):499–505.
74. Halpern AA, Greene R, Nichols T, Burton DS. Compartment syndrome of the interosseous muscles: early recognition and treatment. Clin Orthop Relat Res. 1979;(140):23–5.
75. Allen MJ, Stirling AJ, Crawshaw CV, Barnes MR. Intracompartmental pressure monitoring of leg injuries. An aid to management. J Bone Joint Surg Br. 1985;67(1):53–7.
76. Whitesides TE, Haney TC, Morimoto K, Harada H. Tissue pressure measurements as a determinant for the need of fasciotomy. Clin Orthop Relat Res. 1975;113:43–51.
77. Heppenstall RB, Sapega AA, Scott R, Shenton D, Park YS, Maris J, et al. The compartment syndrome. An experimental and clinical study of muscular energy metabolism using phosphorus nuclear magnetic resonance spectroscopy. Clin Orthop Relat Res. 1988;226:138–55.
78. Heckman MM, Whitesides TE Jr, Grewe SR, Judd RL, Miller M, Lawrence JH III. Histologic determination of the ischemic threshold of muscle in the canine compartment syndrome model. J Orthop Trauma. 1993;7(3):199–210.
79. Brooker AF Jr, Pezeshki C. Tissue pressure to evaluate compartmental syndrome. J Trauma. 1979;19(9):689–91.
80. Ozkayin N, Aktuglu K. Absolute compartment pressure versus differential pressure for the diagnosis of compartment syndrome in tibial fractures. Int Orthop. 2005;29(6):396–401.
81. Janzing HM, Broos PL. Routine monitoring of compartment pressure in patients with tibial fractures: beware of overtreatment! Injury. 2001;32(5):415–21.
82. Hargens AR, Romine JS, Sipe JC, Evans KL, Mubarak SJ, Akeson WH. Peripheral nerve-conduction block by high muscle-compartment pressure. J Bone Joint Surg Am. 1979;61(2):192–200.
83. Heppenstall RB, Sapega AA, Izant T, Fallon R, Shenton D, Park YS, et al. Compartment syndrome: a quantitative study of high-energy phosphorus compounds using 31P-magnetic resonance spectroscopy. J Trauma. 1989;29(8):1113–9.
84. Whitney A, O'Toole RV, Hui E, Sciadini MF, Pollak AN, Manson TT, et al. Do one-time intracompartmental pressure measurements have a high false-positive rate in diagnosing compartment syndrome? J Trauma Acute Care Surg. 2014;76(2):479–83.
85. Kakar S, Firoozabadi R, McKean J, Tornetta P III. Diastolic blood pressure in patients with tibia fractures under anaesthesia: implications for the diagnosis of compartment syndrome. J Orthop Trauma. 2007;21(2):99–103.
86. Shuler FD, Dietz MJ. Physicians' ability to manually detect isolated elevations in leg intracompartmental pressure. J Bone Joint Surg Am. 2010;92(2):361–7.
87. McQueen MM, Duckworth AD, Aitken SA. Court-Brown CM. The estimated sensitivity and specificity of compartment pressure monitoring for acute compartment syndrome. J Bone Joint Surg Am. 2013;95(8):673–7.
88. Badhe S, Baiju D, Elliot R, Rowles J, Calthorpe D. The 'silent' compartment syndrome. Injury. 2009;40(2):220–2.
89. Wright JG, Bogoch ER, Hastings DE. The 'occult' compartment syndrome. J Trauma. 1989;29(1):133–4.
90. Duckworth AD, Mitchell SE, Molyneux SG, White TO, Court-Brown CM, McQueen MM. Acute compartment syndrome of the forearm. J Bone Joint Surg Am. 2012;94(10):e63.
91. Willis RB, Rorabeck CH. Treatment of compartment syndrome in children. Orthop Clin North Am. 1990;21(2):401–12.
92. Shadgan B, Menon M, Sanders D, Berry G, Martin C Jr, Duffy P, et al. Current thinking about acute compartment syndrome of the lower extremity. Can J Surg. 2010;53(5): 329–34.

93. Wall CJ, Richardson MD, Lowe AJ, Brand C, Lynch J, de Steiger RN. Survey of management of acute, traumatic compartment syndrome of the leg in Australia. ANZ J Surg. 2007;77(9):733–7.
94. Williams PR, Russell ID, Mintowt-Czyz WJ. Compartment pressure monitoring--current UK orthopaedic practice. Injury. 1998;29(3):229–32.
95. Mars M, Hadley GP. Raised compartmental pressure in children: a basis for management. Injury. 1998;29(3):183–5.
96. Shadgan B, Menon M, O'Brien PJ, Reid WD. Diagnostic techniques in acute compartment syndrome of the leg. J Orthop Trauma. 2008;22(8):581–7.
97. Arbabi S, Brundage SI, Gentilello LM. Near-infrared spectroscopy: a potential method for continuous, transcutaneous monitoring for compartmental syndrome in critically injured patients. J Trauma. 1999;47(5):829–33.
98. Gentilello LM, Sanzone A, Wang L, Liu PY, Robinson L. Near-infrared spectroscopy versus compartment pressure for the diagnosis of lower extremity compartmental syndrome using electromyography-determined measurements of neuromuscular function. J Trauma. 2001;51(1):1–8, discussion.
99. Shuler MS, Reisman WM, Cole AL, Whitesides TE Jr, Moore TJ. Near-infrared spectroscopy in acute compartment syndrome: case report. Injury. 2011;11
100. Shuler MS, Roskosky M, Kinsey T, Glaser D, Reisman W, Ogburn C, et al. Continual near-infrared spectroscopy monitoring in the injured lower limb and acute compartment syndrome. Bone Joint J. 2018;100-B(6):787–97.
101. Lynch JE, Lynch JK, Cole SL, Carter JA, Hargens AR. Noninvasive monitoring of elevated intramuscular pressure in a model compartment syndrome via quantitative fascial motion. J Orthop Res. 2009;27(4):489–94.
102. Better OS, Zinman C, Reis DN, Har-Shai Y, Rubinstein I, Abassi Z. Hypertonic mannitol ameliorates intracompartmental tamponade in model compartment syndrome in the dog. Nephron. 1991;58(3):344–6.
103. Odland R, Schmidt AH, Hunter B, Kidder L, Bechtold JE, Linzie BM, et al. Use of tissue ultrafiltration for treatment of compartment syndrome: a pilot study using porcine hindlimbs. J Orthop Trauma. 2005;19(4):267–75.
104. Odland RM, Schmidt AH. Compartment syndrome ultrafiltration catheters: report of a clinical pilot study of a novel method for managing patients at risk of compartment syndrome. J Orthop Trauma. 2011;25(6):358–65.
105. Kearns SR, Daly AF, Sheehan K, Murray P, Kelly C, Bouchier-Hayes D. Oral vitamin C reduces the injury to skeletal muscle caused by compartment syndrome. J Bone Joint Surg Br. 2004;86(6):906–11.

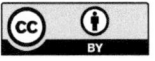

Chapter 6
Limitations of Pressure Measurement

David J. Hak and Cyril Mauffrey

In 1975, Matsen identified increased compartment pressure as the unifying and central pathogenic factor in compartment syndrome [1]. At that same time, Whitesides published a method for tissue pressure measurement [2]. While pressure is an important factor in compartment syndrome, the more important factor is cellular ischemia. Tissue ischemia is the critical factor in compartment syndrome, but at present we do not have a method of assessing the severity and duration of tissue ischemia. Compartment pressure measurement has therefore been used as a surrogate measure of tissue ischemia.

While many clinicians believe the diagnosis of compartment syndrome is a clinical diagnosis based on injury history and physical examination findings, there are circumstances in which compartment pressure measurement is a useful adjunct diagnostic test. These include patients in whom a clinical exam is not feasible or is not reliable such as the unresponsive patient with associated high-risk injuries. Compartment pressure measurement is also typically recommended when a patient's clinical examination findings are unclear. This could include a situation where motor paralysis or sensory changes are present due to a direct nerve injury. Severe and increasing pain is felt to be the most important finding in diagnosing compartment syndrome, but expression of pain severity can vary greatly among patients. Compartment pressure measurement can help rule out compartment syndrome in the patient who expresses an extremely high level of pain despite a clinical scenario of an injury not suspected to result in compartment syndrome.

There are numerous limitations in the use of compartment pressure measurement to diagnose and make treatment decisions in patients at risk for compartment syn-

D. J. Hak (✉)
Hughston Orthopedic Trauma Group, Central Florida Regional Hospital, Sanford, FL, USA

C. Mauffrey
Department of Orthopedic Surgery, Denver Health Medical Center, Denver, CO, USA
e-mail: Cyril.Mauffrey@dhha.org

© The Author(s) 2019
C. Mauffrey et al. (eds.), *Compartment Syndrome*,
https://doi.org/10.1007/978-3-030-22331-1_6

drome. There is no agreement on a specific pressure value for the diagnosis of compartment syndrome. Different tissues and different individuals have a variable response to elevated compartment pressures [3]. Measurement of a single pressure does not allow a clinician to assess the degree of ischemia, since the time course of pressure elevation is unknown. In addition, measurement inaccuracies are common due to technical errors, and pressures can vary greatly based on the location of the measurement with respect to the fracture location. Therefore, most authors indicate that pressure measurements must be correlated with the clinical situation and physical examination findings.

The Problem of Defining a Pressure Measurement Threshold Value

Various absolute pressure measurements were initially recommended as a threshold for the diagnosis of compartment syndrome. In 1978, Mubarak recommended an absolute threshold value of 30 mm Hg [4]. He based this value on the findings that normal muscle capillary pressure is 20–30 mm Hg in cats and dogs, and because clinically pain and paresthesia first appeared around 30 mm Hg in patients undergoing tibial osteotomy. The authors noted that when compartment pressure is >30 mm Hg, capillary pressure is not sufficient to maintain muscle capillary blood flow, stating that, "We believe therefore that it is prudent to use a value close to the capillary blood pressure (20–25 mm Hg) as a criteria for decompression." While the authors recommended 30 mm Hg as a threshold, they did note that there is no single correct pressure for all individuals. They also noted that some of their patients with pressures of 30–40 mm Hg might well have recovered without fasciotomy. They further indicated that, "A spectrum of critical pressure exists depending on many variables, including the measurement technique used."

A higher absolute pressure threshold of 45 mm Hg was suggested by a clinical study of 30 patients at risk for compartment syndrome in which it was noted that all patients who had maximum compartment pressures of 45 mm Hg or less did not require fasciotomy and demonstrated no residual of a missed compartment syndrome at follow-up [5]. The authors noted that, "Perhaps the most significant observation in this series of patients was that individuals varied in their tolerance for increased tissue pressure. Thus, there was a range of intracompartmental pressures in which some patients demonstrated neuromuscular deficits while others did not." The authors indicated that they currently used a tissue pressure in excess of 45 mm Hg as a *relative* indication for surgical decompression, assuming a normal blood pressure, blood volume, and peripheral vascular system, but also noted that these indications must be tempered by the patient's overall condition and the trend of the symptoms, signs, and pressure measurements. The authors highlighted the difficulty in selecting an absolute threshold value for fasciotomy, noting that, "The concept of a critical pressure above which surgical decompression should be performed is of limited value. If a low value is selected as a critical pressure, all patients with significant compartmental syndromes would certainly be included. Yet it is likely that surgery would be performed in a number of patients who would have no significant functional losses without such intervention."

Whitesides introduced the concept of a differential pressure threshold that is widely accepted today. He noted that in the clinical use of pressures, the compartment pressure should be evaluated in association with the patient's diastolic blood pressure [2]. Note that, "Ischemia begins when pressures rises to within 10–30 mm Hg of the diastolic blood pressure. Fasciotomy should usually be performed when the tissue pressure rises to within 10–30 mm Hg of the diastolic pressure in a patient with any of the other signs or symptoms of a compartmental syndrome." This concept of differential threshold helps explain the variable tolerance in absolute pressures noted by other authors. A patient with an elevated diastolic pressure can tolerate a greater elevation in compartment pressure without experiencing ischemia, while a hypotensive patient may develop tissue ischemia with a much lower elevation of their compartment pressure.

McQueen and Court Brown monitored the anterior compartment pressures in a prospective study of 116 patients with tibial fractures using an indwelling slit catheter and followed them to look for sequelae of missed compartment syndrome [6]. Three patients whose differential pressure was <30 mm Hg required a fasciotomy. They reported that had an absolute pressure value of 30 mm Hg been used, 43% of the patients would have had an unnecessary fasciotomy. Using a differential threshold pressure (ΔP) of <30 mm Hg compared to the patient's diastolic blood pressure as the indication for fasciotomy resulted in no cases of missed compartment syndrome. However, the actual duration of the decreased differential threshold pressure in the 3 patients that underwent fasciotomy was not clearly stated. In a larger retrospective series of 850 patients, McQueen and colleagues reported on their use of a differential pressure threshold of <30 mm Hg ($\Delta P < 30$ mm Hg) for greater than 2 hours as the criteria for diagnosis of compartment syndrome [7]. The diagnosis of compartment syndrome was considered to be correct if surgeons noted the escape of muscles at fasciotomy along with muscular color change or necrosis, while they considered the diagnosis of compartment syndrome incorrect if it was possible to primarily close the fasciotomy wounds within 48 hours of the fasciotomy. They calculated that the use of a $\Delta P < 30$ mm Hg for greater than 2 hours has a sensitivity of 94%, a specificity of 98%, a positive predictive value of 93%, and a negative predictive value of 99% for the diagnosis of compartment syndrome [7].

In contrast, Janzing and Broos performed a prospective study of 95 patients in which they measured the anterior compartment pressures for 24 hours in 95 consecutive patients with tibial fractures and followed the patients for 1 year [8]. Eighteen patients were found to have developed compartment syndrome, including 14 patients that underwent fasciotomy and 4 patients that were found to have residual symptoms at follow-up such as toe contractures, hypoesthesia, and muscle weakness. They found wide overlap in the values of the differential pressure between patients with and without the diagnosis of compartment syndrome. While 19% of patients were diagnosed with compartment syndrome, had they used a ΔP of <30 mm Hg, 45.4% of patients would have been diagnosed with compartment syndrome. They found wide overlap in the values of the differential pressure between patients with and without the diagnosis of compartment syndrome. These authors concluded that there did not seem to be a threshold value with an acceptable combination of specificity and sensitivity for the diagnosis of compartment syndrome and cautioned that using a $\Delta P < 30$ mm Hg could result in unnecessary fasciotomies. The authors noted the dilemma faced when identifying a threshold for the diagnosis of compartment syndrome using pressure measurement. They could choose a criterion with high specificity but that would risk missing patients with a compartment syndrome, or they could choose a criterion with high sensitivity which would result in patients undergoing unnecessary fasciotomies.

The Problem of a Single Pressure Measurement

A single measurement of compartment pressure with a single data point provides only limited information. It does not provide information about what the pressure was in prior hours, and it does not predict what the pressure may be during subsequent hours. As such, a single elevated pressure measurement may not accurately reflect the presence or duration of any actual ischemic changes within a compartment.

Investigators studied 46 patients with 48 tibial fractures without clinical suspicion of compartment syndrome and measured pressure in all four compartments after the induction of anesthesia [9]. They did not perform any fasciotomies regardless of the pressure measurements, and at 6 months postoperatively, none of the patients displayed evidence of a missed compartment syndrome. When they compared the compartment pressure measurements with the patient's preoperative diastolic blood pressure, 35% of cases had a $\Delta P < 30$ mm Hg. Twenty-four percent of cases had a $\Delta P < 20$ mm Hg, and 22% had absolute pressure > 45 mm Hg, yet none of these patients underwent fasciotomy and none developed sequela of a missed compartment syndrome. These investigators concluded that a one-time measurement of compartment pressure overestimates the rate of compartment syndrome and may lead to unnecessary fasciotomy. Using the criteria of $\Delta P < 30$ mm Hg in patients without clinical symptoms to diagnose compartment syndrome would lead to a 35% false-positive rate.

O'Toole and colleagues have reported a wide variation in the rate of diagnosis and treatment of compartment syndrome among academic traumatologists practicing at the same level I trauma center [10]. In a review of 386 patients with tibia fractures, the diagnosis of compartment syndrome between different surgeons ranged from 2% to 24% ($p < 0.005$). Equally noteworthy was that a similar variation was seen in the surgeon's use of compartment pressure measurement, which seemed to approximately parallel their rate of compartment syndrome diagnosis. While this study did not examine the medicolegal aspects of compartment syndrome, there is a general sense that once compartment pressures are measured, there is a low threshold for proceeding with a fasciotomy.

The Problems of Measurement Accuracy

Numerous studies have examined the accuracy of compartment pressure measurement. These studies have examined the type of needle used, the technique, and the location of pressure measurement.

Investigators compared three types of needles in a canine mode of acute compartment syndrome [11]. Needles tested included a standard end bore needle, a side-posted needle, and a slit catheter. A concern regarding the use of a standard bore needle is that a soft tissue plug within the needle can prevent accurate pressure measurement. They found no statistical difference between slit catheter and side-ported needle. However, standard end bore needle measurements were consistently higher than the other two methods ($p < 0.001$).

Overestimation of compartment pressure measurements with standard end bore needles was also confirmed in another study [12]. This study, which compared use of a commercial pressure monitor (Stryker, Mahwah, NJ), arterial line monitor, and the technique using IV tubing as described by Whitesides, found that the Whitesides technique had the highest standard errors and provided clinically unacceptable scatter in its measurements.

Dr. Whitesides rebutted the reported unacceptable reliability with a standard bevel-tipped needle and the Whitesides technique, stating that this finding was contrary to his cumulative clinical and research experience. He indicated that when properly used with a small required saline flush to assure a fluid continuum between tissue and the pressure monitor, this technique had acceptable accuracy [13]. They performed simultaneous testing of three different devices (slit catheters, side ported needles, and standard 18-gauge end bore bevel-tipped needles) in the same area of fusiform muscle against increasing intramuscular pressure using the same transducer and monitor and reported that the side-ported needle, slit catheter, and standard 18-gauge bevel-tipped needle were statistically equivalent.

In his original description of compartment pressure measurement, Whitesides used a 1.25 mm capillary tube, while current technique typically uses IV tubing that has an internal diameter of 3 mm. This difference in diameter makes it more difficult to differentiate a flat versus a convex versus a concave fluid meniscus during the pressure measurement. when using the 3 mm internal diameter IV tubing. If an electronic transducer is not available for pressure measurement, Whitesides and colleagues recommended averaging several consecutive saline measurements.

Investigators have also highlighted technical problems associated with the measurement of compartment pressures [14]. In this study, a consistent model of lower leg compartment syndrome was created in cadaveric specimens. Thirty-eight physicians, including residents, fellows, and attending physicians, were observed while they measured the four compartments of the lower leg using a commercial compartment pressure measurement device. Only 31% of the measurements were performed using the correct technique. In 39% of the measurements, there were minor errors in the technique. Minor errors included failure to maintain the angle of insertion after zeroing, failure to use the proper amount of saline for flushing, and inconsistent zeroing between each measurement. In the remaining 30% of measurements, participants made catastrophic errors. These included failure to properly assemble the components of the monitor, not flushing the air from the syringe/transducer apparatus, failure to zero the monitor before insertion, zeroing the monitor under the skin, and failure to insert the needle into the correct anatomic space.

Of the 31% of measurements performed using the correct technique, only 60% were with 5 m Hg of the known compartment pressure. Of the 39% of measurements made with minor errors in technique, only 42% were with 5 m Hg of the known compartment pressure. Of the 30% of measurements made with catastrophic errors, only 22% were with 5 m Hg of the known compartment pressure.

The investigators concluded that errors are common in compartment pressure measurement. While proper technique improved accuracy, only 60% of these measurements were with 5 m Hg of the known compartment pressure. Given their findings, the investigators cautioned that measurement accuracy should not be assumed and reported measurements viewed as within a range of values rather than as an absolute value.

Another group of investigators compared three measurement methods in 26 patients with suspected compartment syndrome, measuring 97 muscle compartments in 31 injured limbs. The measurement methods used were a modification of Whitesides' needle manometer technique using a straight 18-gauge needle with a central venous pressure monitor, an electronic transducer-tipped catheter (Depuy Synthes, West Chester, PA), and a solid-state transducer intracompartmental catheter (Stryker, Mahwah NJ) [15]. The overall intraclass correlation coefficient for the three methods was 0.83 (range 0.77–0.88), indicating only satisfactory agreement. The mean difference among measurements in each compartment was 8.3 mm Hg (range 0–51 mm Hg), while 27% showed major differences that exceeded 10 mm Hg. The authors concluded that the methods were similar but not completely reliable for measuring compartment pressure. They emphasized that while all methods appeared useful as aids in diagnosis of compartment syndrome, compartment pressure data, especially single readings, must be interpreted in view of clinical findings. They recommended that no single pressure measurement be used as the primary determinant in individual decisions for or against fasciotomy and emphasized that specific values must be considered in the context of the patients' overall clinical picture.

Another factor that influences the measured compartment pressure value is the location of the measurement with respect to the fracture. Compartment pressures were measured at the level of the fracture and at 5 cm increments proximally and distally in 25 consecutive patients with closed tibial fractures [16]. The peak compartment pressure was usually found at the level of the fracture and was always located within 5 cm of the fracture site. The measured pressures decreased progressively at increasing distances proximal and distal to the site of the highest pressure measurement. Most notably, decreases of 20 mm Hg were common just 5 cm adjacent to the site of the highest pressure measurement.

References

1. Matsen FA 3rd. Compartment syndrome: an unified concept. Clin Orthop Relat Res. 1975;113:8–14.
2. Whitesides TE Jr, Haney TC, Morimoto K, Harada H. Tissue pressure measurements as a determinant for the need of fasciotomy. Clin Orthop Relat Res. 1975;113:43–51.
3. Matsen FA 3rd, Mayo KA, Krugmire RB Jr, Sheridan GW, Kraft GH. A model compartmental syndrome in man with particular reference to the quantification of nerve function. J Bone Joint Surg Am. 1977;59:648–53.
4. Mubarak SJ, Owen CA, Hargens AR, Garetto LP, Akeson WH. Acute compartment syndromes: diagnosis and treatment with the aid of the wick catheter. J Bone Joint Surg Am. 1978;60:1091–5.
5. Matsen FA 3rd, Winquist RA, Krugmire RB Jr. Diagnosis and management of compartmental syndromes. J Bone Joint Surg Am. 1980;62:286–91.
6. McQueen MM, Court-Brown CM. Compartment monitoring in tibial fractures. The pressure threshold for decompression. J Bone Joint Surg Br. 1996;78:99–104.
7. McQueen MM, Duckworth AD, Aitken SA, Court-Brown CM. The estimated sensitivity and specificity of compartment pressure monitoring for acute compartment syndrome. J Bone Joint Surg Am. 2013;95:673–7.
8. Janzing HM, Broos PL. Routine monitoring of compartment pressure in patients with tibial fractures: beware of overtreatment! Injury. 2001;32:415–21.
9. Whitney A, O'Toole RV, Hui E, Sciadini MF, Pollak AN, Manson TT, Eglseder WA, Andersen RC, Lebrun C, Doro C, Nascone JW. Do one-time intracompartmental pressure measurements have a high false-positive rate in diagnosing compartment syndrome? J Trauma Acute Care Surg. 2014;76:479–83.
10. O'Toole RV, Whitney A, Merchant N, Hui E, Higgins J, Kim TT, Sagebien C. Variation in diagnosis of compartment syndrome by surgeons treating tibial shaft fractures. J Trauma. 2009;67:735–41.
11. Moed BR, Thorderson PK. Measurement of intracompartmental pressure: a comparison of the slit catheter, side-ported needle, and simple needle. J Bone Joint Surg Am. 1993;75:231–5.
12. Boody AR, Wongworawat MD. Accuracy in the measurement of compartment pressures: a comparison of three commonly used devices. J Bone Joint Surg Am. 2005;87:2415–22.
13. Hammerberg EM, Whitesides TE, Seiler JG. The reliability of measurement of tissue pressure in compartment syndrome. J Orthop Trauma. 2012;26:24–31.
14. Large TM, Agel J, Holtzman DJ, Benirschke SK, Krieg JC. Interobserver variability in the measurement of lower leg compartment pressures. J Orthop Trauma. 2015;29:316–21.
15. Collinge C, Kuper M. Comparison of three methods for measuring intracompartmental pressure in injured limbs of trauma patients. J Orthop Trauma. 2010;24:364–8.
16. Heckman MM, Whitesides TE Jr, Grewe SR, Rooks MD. Compartment pressure in association with closed tibial fractures: the relationship between tissue pressure, compartment, and the distance from the site of the fracture. J Bone Joint Surg Am. 1994;76:1285–92.

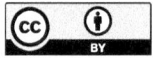

Chapter 7
Fasciotomy: Upper Extremity

Kyros Ipaktchi, Jessica Wingfield, and Salih Colakoglu

Background

- Early fasciotomy is the standard of care for upper extremity compartment syndrome (UECS) and may prevent the development of irreversible contractures of forearm and hand musculature, a pathology initially described by Volkmann [1]. Compartment syndrome (CS) is a feared orthopedic complication and a common cause for permanent functional damage and limb loss as well as one of the most common causes for litigation in orthopedic surgery [2, 3].
- CS of the forearm is the second most common cause of CS in the extremities given the injury proneness of the upper extremity and hand as a prime organ of prehension and grasp [4]. Given this important physiologic function, one can argue that the functional loss due to an established CS is higher than that of the lower extremity.
- For UECS, a high level of alertness to clinical symptoms such as pain to passive stretch and increasing pain or analgesic requirements is key to not miss the diagnosis in the alert patient.
- UECS shares common etiologies for CS seen in other body areas: either an external reduction of CS size such as external pressure from casts, dressings, and gravity or increase in compartmental size as seen in bleeding and fracture displacement, microvascular barrier damage in ischemia, burn injury, and envenom-

K. Ipaktchi (✉)
Orthopedic Department, Denver Health Medical Center, Denver, CO, USA
e-mail: kyros.ipaktchi@dhha.org

J. Wingfield
Orthopedic Department, University of Colorado, Aurora, CO, USA

S. Colakoglu
Plastic Surgery Department, University of Colorado, Aurora, CO, USA
e-mail: salih.colakoglu@ucdenver.edu

© The Author(s) 2019
C. Mauffrey et al. (eds.), *Compartment Syndrome*,
https://doi.org/10.1007/978-3-030-22331-1_7

ations [4]. Several additional etiologies are pertinent to UECS such as iatrogenic extravasations of intravenous fluids, upper extremity arterial catheterizations [5], and electrical trauma [6].

- UECS is most commonly encountered in the forearm, which has three designated compartments (i.e., the lateral (mobile wad), the dorsal extensor, and the volar) of which contains the bulk of muscle mass in the flexor compartment. There are ten designated hand compartments which can be affected in hand compartment syndrome as seen, for instance, in crushing injuries (exploded hand syndrome), fractures and dislocations, as well as extravasations.
- When performing fasciotomies for UECS, special emphasis must be placed to decompress the muscles of the deep flexor compartment due to their non-redundant blood supply which makes them especially prone to ischemic damage [7].

Recommendations

Pathophysiology

Compartment Syndrome is a result of tissue ischemia which arises from a reduction of the pressure gradient between the vascular bed and the surrounding soft tissues which can become pressurized due to intracompartmental pressure rise or external pressure [8].

The severity of a CS has been described by several authors as dependent on time and amount of pressure as well as the degree of tissue injury [4]. Recommendations are to differentiate separate phases of CS, which may help guide treatment [4]. As such, pending nonestablished CS can be differentiated from the acute, reversible CS (within 8 hrs of trauma), and acute irreversible CS (later than 8 hrs). This is separated from late established CS and even later in the upper extremity Volkmann's contracture as a sequelae of CS. Independent from these acute traumatic conditions, chronic exertional CS can be seen as its own entity with different treatment modalities.

Diagnosis

Given the importance of early intervention before irreversible damage has incurred, the diagnosis of CS in the upper extremity relies primarily on the recognition of clinical scenarios where a CS can be expected in combination with detection of early clinical signs such as pain to stretch – increasing pain out of proportion and increased analgesic needs. The classic signs of compartment syndrome ("5 or 6 Ps") included late irreversible changes and are not recommended in diagnosing early compartment syndrome [9].

Pressure measurements – especially in the obtunded patient – remain an important adjunct to CS diagnosis. The absolute pressure theory as described by Matsen has been replaced by differential pressure models in which fasciotomy is indicated when the delta pressure, measured as the difference between the compartmental pressures and arterial or venous blood pressures, falls to 30 and 20 mmHg, respectively [10].

When using pressure measurement devices, the higher accuracy of side port or slit catheters as compared to straight catheters has been pointed out [11]. In addition, it was shown that pressures measured within a single compartment can vary significantly with regard to distance to fracture site [12]. So standardization of measurement methods and sites is recommended for repeat measurements. With regard to the most commonly affected deep flexor compartments in UECS, safe techniques for pressure measurement have been described [13].

Treatment

Close observation with documented hourly repeat exams of a patient with concerns for a pending CS is mandatory. This includes removing all constrictive dressings and tight splints. As the provision of tissue oxygenation is key to prevention of a CS, medical optimization of a patient is of paramount importance. This includes full resuscitation, optimization of blood pressure and oxygenation, as well as keeping the extremity at slight elevation (heart level). Further elevation will reduce perfusion pressures, reduce differential pressures, and thereby increase tissue damage.

If medical optimization is unsuccessful or the patient presents with an acute CS, fasciotomy must be performed as emergent procedure to decompress tissues and salvage tissue function.

General recommendations for the upper extremity are similar to concepts of fasciotomy elsewhere in the body in that surgical decompression must be performed through adequate incisions which parallel the length of the fasciotomy incisions. Care must be taken not to add morbidity by injuring cutaneous branches in the forearm (e.g., MABC/LABC) and to decompress all components of the compartment. Given the importance of maintaining joint motion in the upper extremities and protecting important neurovascular bundles which could be exposed by nonjudicious incisions, recommendations are to perform curvilinear incisions and to avoid crossing flexion creases in a straight fashion.

At the brachium level, three compartments are described: the volar (anterior) compartment containing the biceps and brachialis and coracobrachialis, which is released through an anterior or anterolateral approach, the posterior compartment with the three heads of the triceps, and the deltoid compartment – the latter two can be decompressed through a posterolateral approach taking care to release the tight epimysium of the deltoid compartment.

In the more common forearm compartment syndrome, care must be taken to decompress both the superficial and deep components of the volar flexor compartment. This includes the investing fascia of individual fascial compartments in the deep flexor muscles (PQ, FDP, FPL). Proximally, the lacertus fibrosus must be released as a possible site of compression as well as distally the carpal tunnel. The dorsal extensor compartment is approached through a dorsal midline straight incision – the mobile wad can usually be released via either the volar or dorsal approaches.

When releasing the forearm, consideration to progressive swelling-induced exposure of released neurovascular bundles must be taken into account. While the standard extended Henry type of release with Brunner style zigzag extension into the carpal tunnel and antecubital fossa may be adequate, flap creating exposures which maximize a radial-based forearm flap and ulnar to radial dissection across the flexor crease of the wrist may optimize median nerve coverage as well as preserve the option for later radial artery-based flap coverage in complex soft tissue defects of the hand. Specific injury patterns such as burn or electrical trauma may need additional release of eschar and neurovascular bundles.

For compartment syndromes of the hand and fingers, standardized incisions are necessary to minimize morbidity given the tight skin envelope and complex anatomical content of these compartments. On the volar side, longitudinal incisions paralleling the radial and ulnar border of thenar and hypothenar eminences are described to optimize the release of these muscle compartments and protect neurovascular bundles. Commonly, carpal tunnel releases for UECS are performed as extensile approaches to connect to the forearm fasciotomy but can also be done in isolation, in which case the carpal tunnel must be released 4–5 cm into the volar forearm fascia. On the dorsal side, the release of the interosseous spaces is usually performed via two longitudinal incisions overlying the first and second as well as third and fourth interosseous spaces. These incisions parallel the metacarpal shafts, and care must be taken to preserve a wide enough skin bridge. When releasing finger compartments, additional morbidity by accidentally damaging dominant sensory nerves must be avoided. As such, radial incisions are performed on the thumb and index finger and ulnar incisions on the index long and ring fingers. These unilateral, midaxial incisions traverse the Cleland ligament – the dorsal roof of the neurovascular bundle – and thus release compression around these structures.

After fasciotomies for UECS, special care must be taken to ensure functional rehabilitation is started soon. This includes splinting the extremity (especially hand) in a functional position in the operating room and starting with early therapy including edema care and coverage once second look procedures confirm a viable wound bed [14]. Early coverage of important functional units takes precedent and can include flap and/or skin graft coverage as well as dynamic wound closure techniques. In all instances, the creation of a secondary iatrogenic compartment syndrome by overly tight closing compartments must be excluded [6].

Limitations and Pitfalls

Unfortunately, the correct diagnosis and early treatment of every CS at a function recoverable stage appears to be still an elusive target. This may be explained by the complex multifactorial etiology of CS and the progressive nature of the disease which can be easily missed unless there is accurate documentation and standardized handover between care teams.

The fear of delayed fasciotomies and the possible risk of adverse outcomes to patients as well as litigation to institution and provider may result in an overly broad indication of fasciotomies which if done improperly can add significant morbidity to an already traumatized limb [15]. This concern may be especially applicable to the noncooperative, obtunded patient as well as in the young pediatric populations where it may be difficult to elicit clinical signs of CS. It is not surprising that especially in the pediatric patient population, there is a higher rate of plaintiff verdicts [2].

From a legal perspective, one of the main concerns and causes for successful plaintiff verdicts in the treatment of CS appears to be a late release of an established CS defined as later than 8 hrs post documentation of a CS [16]. At this point, it becomes easier for the plaintiff counsel to argue that the incurred damage was due to the late intervention and independent of a prior trauma [2]. While late intervention is a common pitfall seen in CS, also in the upper extremity, a common pitfall lies in the inadequate release of a CS. This can be seen in failure to release adjacent structures which can be affected by CS – here the incomplete release of neurovascular bundles in the AC fossa and carpal tunnel need to be stressed. Also the failure to completely release deep flexor compartments in the forearm and inadequate incisions across flexor creases commonly result in avoidable morbidity. Of special legal concern is the occurrence of an iatrogenic CS, which in the setting of an upper extremity surgery can be seen after tight fascial closures of forearm fractures or attempts of early closure of fasciotomy incisions. The release of established and irreversible CS is associated with high infection rates and limb loss and does not add benefit [17]. Here consideration for a midterm release of forearm and hand contractures should take precedent [18].

Future Directions

While fasciotomies appear to remain the standard surgical treatment for established CS, standardization of technique to minimize morbidity is an ongoing effort.

Future research is directed at improving diagnostic tools and minimizing delays in treatment as well as optimizing wound care to facilitate early closure to prevent secondary limb injuries [19].

Similar to the active research of breakthrough pain in cancer patient care [20], a future research direction may be aimed toward improved and possibly automated detection of inadequate analgesia as an early sign of evolving CS. Going one step further, earlier research demonstrated that predictive algorithms can be developed to alert clinicians to the heightened risk for developing a CS [21] in patients with specific injury diagnosis and scenarios such as increased blood loss, vascular injury, and open fractures. While this may seem trivial to the specialized clinician, missed compartment syndromes continue to occur, and every option to prevent these should be utilized.

There is ongoing research into the development of improved pressure sensors as well as combined sensors for tissue pH, muscle microvascular blood flow, and oxygenation [22–24]. This includes measuring perfusion pressure with photoplethysmography and near-infrared spectroscopy-pH probes [23]. An interesting novel but experimental method is the use of ultrafiltration catheters to measure in real time the accumulation of muscle injury markers such as CK and LDH [25].

It appears possible that advances in these different diagnostic avenues can improve our skills in rapid detection and treatment of the CS at an early stage.

Take-Home Message

- Surgeon must be alert to possible development of a compartment syndrome even before clinical symptoms have set in and in certain circumstances perform prophylactic fasciotomies (high energy segmental fractures, ischemia-reperfusion trauma, obtunded patients).
- The deep flexor muscles of the forearm are especially injury prone to ischemia and compressive damage due to more limited vascular supply (angiosome concept) and separate investing fascia.
- In electric trauma and burn injury, perform separate release of neurovascular structures and constricting eschar.
- Any diagnosed CS needs emergent fasciotomy. This procedure must be performed in a standardized way to protect key functional structures (e.g., NV bundles, tendons, and joints). In the upper extremity, special care must be taken to protect these structures from prolonged exposure and secondary compression due to swelling of fasciotomy flaps or compression from unreleased fascial septal structures including the bicipital aponeurosis.
- Early functional rehabilitation including splinting and compression therapy is essential in the treatment of upper extremity compartment syndrome and must start after fasciotomy.
- Communication of all team members nursing staff, resident team, and provider is essential to avoid delay in care. All findings must be documented and closely monitored in cases of suspected but not established compartment syndromes.

References

1. VOLKMAN & R. Die ischaemischen Muskellahmungen und Kontrakturen. Centralblat fur hirurgie.1881;8:801–803.
2. DePasse JM, et al. Assessment of malpractice claims associated with acute compartment syndrome. J Am Acad Orthop Surg. 2017;25:e109–13.
3. Marchesi M, et al. A sneaky surgical emergency: acute compartment syndrome. Retrospective analysis of 66 closed claims, medico-legal pitfalls and damages evaluation. Injury. 2014;45(Suppl 6):S16–20.
4. Leversedge FJ, Moore TJ, Peterson BC, Seiler JG 3rd. Compartment syndrome of the upper extremity. J Hand Surg Am. 2011;36:544–59; quiz 560.

5. Omori S, et al. Compartment syndrome of the arm caused by transcatheter angiography or angioplasty. Orthopedics. 2013;36:e121–5.

6. Lee DH, Desai MJ, Gauger EM. Electrical injuries of the hand and upper extremity. J Am Acad Orthop Surg. 2018; https://doi.org/10.5435/JAAOS-D-17-00833.

7. Inoue Y, Taylor GI. The angiosomes of the forearm: anatomic study and clinical implications. Plast Reconstr Surg. 1996;98:195–210.

8. Prasarn ML, Ouellette EA. Acute compartment syndrome of the upper extremity. J Am Acad Orthop Surg. 2011;19:49–58.

9. Matsen FA 3rd, Krugmire RB Jr. Compartmental syndromes. Surg Gynecol Obstet. 1978;147:943–9.

10. Whitesides TE Jr, Haney TC, Harada H, Holmes HE, Morimoto K. A simple method for tissue pressure determination. Arch Surg. 1975;110:1311–3.

11. Boody AR, Wongworawat MD. Accuracy in the measurement of compartment pressures: a comparison of three commonly used devices. J Bone Joint Surg Am. 2005;87:2415–22.

12. Heckman MM, Whitesides TE Jr, Grewe SR, Rooks MD. Compartment pressure in association with closed tibial fractures. The relationship between tissue pressure, compartment, and the distance from the site of the fracture. J Bone Joint Surg Am. 1994;76:1285–92.

13. McCarthy DM, Sotereanos DG, Towers JD, Britton CA, Herndon JH. A cadaveric and radiologic assessment of catheter placement for the measurement of forearm compartment pressures. Clin Orthop Relat Res. 1995:266–70.

14. Kamolz L-P, Kitzinger HB, Karle B, Frey M. The treatment of hand burns. Burns. 2009;35:327–37.

15. Lagerstrom CF, Reed RL 2nd, Rowlands BJ, Fischer RP. Early fasciotomy for acute clinically evident posttraumatic compartment syndrome. Am J Surg. 1989;158:36–9.

16. Bhattacharyya T, Vrahas MS. The medical-legal aspects of compartment syndrome. J Bone Joint Surg Am. 2004;86-A:864–8.

17. Ritenour AE, et al. Complications after fasciotomy revision and delayed compartment release in combat patients. J Trauma. 2008;64:S153–61; discussion S161–2.

18. Stevanovic M, Sharpe F. Late management of compartment syndrome. In: Abzug JM, Kozin SH, Zlotolow DA, editors. The pediatric upper extremity. New York: Springer; 2015. p. 1453–78.

19. Shirley ED, Mai V, Neal KM, Kiebzak GM. Wound closure expectations after fasciotomy for paediatric compartment syndrome. J Child Orthop. 2018;12:9–14.

20. O'Hagan P, Mercadante S. Breakthrough cancer pain: the importance of the right treatment at the right time. Eur J Pain. 2018;22:1362–74.

21. Kim JYS, et al. A prognostic model for the risk of development of upper extremity compartment syndrome in the setting of brachial artery injury. Ann Plast Surg. 2009;62:22–7.

22. Schmidt AH, et al. Continuous near-infrared spectroscopy demonstrates limitations in monitoring the development of acute compartment syndrome in patients with leg injuries. J Bone Joint Surg Am. 2018;100:1645–52.

23. Challa ST, Hargens AR, Uzosike A, Macias BR. Muscle microvascular blood flow, oxygenation, pH, and perfusion pressure decrease in simulated acute compartment syndrome. J Bone Joint Surg Am. 2017;99:1453–9.

24. Weick JW, et al. Direct measurement of tissue oxygenation as a method of diagnosis of acute compartment syndrome. J Orthop Trauma. 2016;30:585–91.

25. Odland RM, Schmidt AH. Compartment syndrome ultrafiltration catheters: report of a clinical pilot study of a novel method for managing patients at risk of compartment syndrome. J Orthop Trauma. 2011;25:358–65.

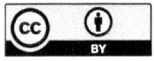

Chapter 8
Compartment Syndrome of the Lower Extremity

Cody M. Tillinghast and Joshua L. Gary

Introduction

Acute compartment syndrome is a surgical emergency that can threaten life and the limb. Moreover, lower extremity compartment syndrome is most commonly associated with high-energy mechanisms of injury; however, a high index of suspicion should be maintained with low-energy or penetrating trauma, vascular or crush injuries, and prolonged periods of immobility. Rare presentations are even documented in association with diabetes mellitus, hypothyroidism, malignancy, viral-induced myositis, nephrotic syndrome, and bleeding disorders [1]. Most practitioners associate lower extremity compartment syndrome with the leg, but other sites including the buttock, thigh, and foot can develop the same pathology. Serial physical examinations by an experienced provider remain the best tool for accurate diagnosis, while intramuscular compartment pressure measurements are best used as an adjunct especially when a complete physical examination is not possible. Compartment syndrome, unlike many musculoskeletal conditions, is much easier to treat than to accurately diagnose. Prompt fasciotomies with release of all involved muscular compartments prevent the life- and limb-threatening sequelae of a missed compartment syndrome. Although fasciotomies are associated with increased blood loss and elevated risk of infection and commonly require split-thickness skin grafts in lieu of closure, they prevent irreversible ischemic tissue loss and potential for lifetime disability. We hope the reader uses this chapter to assist in diagnosis and treatment of patients with potential compartment syndrome.

Electronic Supplementary Material The online version of this chapter (https://doi.org/10.1007/978-3-030-22331-1_8) contains supplementary material, which is available to authorized users.

C. M. Tillinghast (✉) · J. L. Gary
University of Texas Health Science Center at Houston, McGovern Medical School,
Department of Orthopedic Surgery, Houston, TX, USA
e-mail: Cody.M.Tillinghast@uth.tmc.edu; Joshua.L.Gary@uth.tmc.edu

© The Author(s) 2019
C. Mauffrey et al. (eds.), *Compartment Syndrome*,
https://doi.org/10.1007/978-3-030-22331-1_8

Pathophysiology

Compartment syndrome is the result of fascial compartment pressures surpassing perfusion pressure, causing tissue ischemia and eventual necrosis [2]. After a local insult, traumatic or others, volume increases to a compartment from bleeding or inflammation, leading to the onset of local tissue edema as a result. Fascial compartments in the body have finite volumes with limited ability for elastic expansion, so pressure levels correspondingly increase. Heightened tissue pressure corresponds with an increase in venous pressure, thus decreasing the arteriovenous gradient. As this gradient decreases, microvascular flow through capillaries falls, and inadequate perfusion of the tissue eventually results, causing ischemic changes to the tissues. Permanent damage to muscle tissue may result shortly after 4–8 hours of ischemia [3, 4]. Anoxic damage to endothelial cells results in further increases to vessel wall permeability that, along with decreased venous outflow, perpetuates the local edema and pressure increases. Eventual muscle necrosis leads to the release of myoglobin into the blood with associated metabolic acidosis and hyperkalemia. Severity is based on extent of muscle compartments involved and duration of the ischemic changes. The worst of cases may potentiate cardiac arrhythmias, renal failure, shock, or hypothermia. Fasciotomies remove the volume limitations to the compartment, drastically altering the pressure gradients with the goal of restoring tissue perfusion.

Medical Management and Missed Compartment Syndromes

All patients presenting after high-energy mechanisms of injury should be promptly evaluated using Advanced Trauma Life Support (ATLS) protocols to identify and treat life-threatening injuries [5]. Patients presenting after prolonged immobilization should be evaluated according to their signs and symptoms. Ischemic reperfusion events can occur following vascular injuries or prolonged compression events. Bywater's or crush syndrome is a traumatic rhabdomyolysis where cellular necrosis from a crush injury results in increased serum myoglobin and potassium, leading to acidosis and kidney failure [6]. Fluid resuscitation with consideration of added sodium bicarbonate helps to dilute increased myoglobin and urea concentrations from muscle necrosis and counteract the associated metabolic acidosis, thereby limiting acute tubular necrosis and renal dysfunction [6].

A Foley catheter is recommended to ensure adequate fluid resuscitation and monitor renal failure. Dark, tea-colored urine is suggestive of myoglobinuria and ongoing rhabdomyolysis [6]. Serial serum myoglobin levels may also be of benefit for diagnosis and guidance of need for ongoing fluid resuscitation [7]. Myoglobin levels may be elevated in trauma patients without acute compartment syndrome, especially those with muscle injury at multiple sites throughout the body. Increasing levels of myoglobin with declining renal function should alert the provider that muscle necrosis is ongoing and prompt fasciotomy with debridement of necrotic muscle, while decreasing myoglobin levels can be reassuring to the provider.

A type and screen for potential blood transfusion is recommended as patients who undergo fasciotomy often bleed from the injured tissues, open wounds, and/or negative pressure wound therapy (NPWT). Blood transfusion should also be an early component of the resuscitation of the trauma patient in shock [8].

Missed compartment syndromes provide a treatment conundrum for the surgeon as opening a closed necrotic compartment may introduce a significant risk for deep infection and its sequelae. These are usually patients who have had ongoing pain for several hours that spontaneously resolves without fasciotomy. Neurologic and potential vascular compromise results in soft tissue death and potential limb loss. However, it is difficult for the surgeon to know if some muscle in the compartment can be salvaged without direct intraoperative examination of the muscle. Computed tomography (CT) scanning provides soft tissue windows that might alert the surgeon for any abnormalities in the musculature and the extent of myonecrosis. Worsening renal function, despite adequate fluid resuscitation, also forces the surgeon's hand toward fasciotomy for debridement of necrotic musculature which is a source of myoglobin, potassium, and tissue thromboplastin [6]. Complications as a result can vary based on the extent of necrosis but can include cardiotoxicity, disseminated intravascular coagulation, renal failure, and sepsis, leading to multiorgan failure or death. Observation without fasciotomy should be reserved for patients without signs of sepsis or worsening renal function that present to the surgeon with no ongoing pain.

Intracompartmental Pressure Measurements and Continuous Monitoring

The use of intracompartmental pressure measurements and continuous monitoring remains controversial. For the awake and alert patient, serial physical examinations remain the best diagnostic methods with the "one P," pain, being the hallmark symptom of compartment syndrome. An awake and alert patient with signs and symptoms of compartment syndrome concerning enough to undergo pressure measurements should probably just be taken to the operating room for emergent fasciotomy.

Intracompartmental pressure monitoring is especially useful in patients obtunded due to illicit substances or traumatic brain injuries; however, these measurements remain imperfect and lack specificity. Measurements can be made with commercially available devices with a side-port needle catheter or with an arterial line setup [9]. Thresholds for absolute pressure and ΔP (diastolic blood pressure – absolute compartment pressure) have been set to prevent any missed compartment syndrome but may lead to unnecessary fasciotomy in many patients. In a prospective study, patients with tibia fractures undergoing planned intramedullary nailing were evaluated with four compartment preoperative pressure measurements. There was no clinical suspicion for compartment syndrome for any of these patients up to the time of surgery. However, measurements meeting an accepted threshold for fasciotomy at absolute pressure $>= 40$ mm Hg or $\Delta P <= 30$ mmHg were present in 35% of patients. These patients were followed for 6 months with no signs of missed compartment syndrome [10]. This point is reiterated in another prospective study of diaphyseal tibia fractures with continuous pressure monitoring where an absolute pressure threshold of 30 mmHg or 40 mmHg would have led to 43% and 23% of unnecessary fasciotomies, respectively. This study recommended the $\Delta P <= 30$mmHg as the best indication for fasciotomy and also highlighted one-time measurements do not preclude subsequent development of a compartment syndrome [11]. Continuous monitoring may address this limitation but requires many hospital resources that may include an intensive care or intermediate care bed and may not change the ultimate outcomes. Challenges with pressure measurements include low adherence to proper technique and substantial decreases in accuracy of measurement even with small errors in technique [12]. Overall, intracompartmental pressure monitoring should not be used not only as a screening tool but also to give evidence to confirm clinical suspicion as needed [2].

Gluteal Compartment Syndrome

The gluteal region is a rare anatomic location for the development of compartment syndrome. Most cases will result from prolonged immobilization secondary to heavy drug/alcohol use or surgical positioning [13]. Thorough examination of all extremities should be performed in patients presenting to the hospital after prolonged immobilization. These patients may be obtunded secondary to alcohol and illicit drug use or potentially due to neurodegenerative disorders, thereby limiting a full history and physical examination. Prolonged surgeries in the lateral decubitus or lithotomy are the most implicated surgical positions, causing a gluteal compartment syndrome [14]. Traumatic injury and gluteal compartment syndrome comprise approximately 20% of cases [13]. These usually result from a crushing mechanism to the lower lumbar spine, pelvis, and buttocks area. Prolonged extrication time and/or crushing mechanism with heavy objects should alert the provider for any potential development. Additional causes may include vascular injury, epidural analgesia after total hip arthroplasty, anticoagulation, overuse or exertion, and necrotizing fasciitis infections [13]. The gluteal compartment syndrome is also frequently associated with the previously discussed crush syndrome, so holistic management to prevent renal failure and systemic complications of rhabdomyolysis is of paramount importance.

There are three compartments in the gluteal region: tensor fasciae latae (TFL), gluteus medius and minimus, and gluteus maximus. The gluteus maximus is the largest of the three and supplied by the inferior gluteal nerve and vessels. This muscle is the main extensor and external rotator of the leg, originating on the posterior ilium and dorsal sacrum extending over the gluteus medius to join the posterior iliotibial tract. Deep and superolateral to the maximus resides the gluteus medius muscle. The medius originates on the ilium and inserts on the greater trochanter overlaying the gluteus minimus. The superior gluteal nerve and vessels supply the gluteus medius and minimus, and these muscles together form a single compartment lying between the maximus and TFL. The TFL is in its own compartment that originates on anterior iliac crest and anterior superior iliac spine blending distally with the iliotibial band in the proximal thigh. Although not directly contained within these compartments, the sciatic nerve is at risk for a compressive neuropathy due to excessive swelling of the gluteal muscles or traumatic hematoma [14].

Alert patients will present with severe pain in the gluteal regions and may complain of lower extremity paresthesias. Physical examination will reveal tense and painful buttocks to touch, possibly ecchymoses, and/or Morel-Lavallee lesions. Passive motion of adduction and flexion of the hip would exacerbate pain in the examinable patient as it counters the typical movements of the gluteal musculature decreasing compartment volumes.

As gluteal compartment syndrome is rare and examinations are occasionally limited, the surgeon may choose to use intracompartmental pressure measurements more frequently than other locations in the lower extremity. Optimal needle placement for compartment pressure measurements was studied using cadavers and found to be clear of neurovascular bundles [14]. The gluteus maximus needle should be placed 2 cm inferior and lateral to the posterior superior iliac spine. Advance the needle until contact of the iliac wing and withdraw approximately 4 mm to assure localization within the muscle belly. The needle directed toward the medius/minimus compartment is placed 2 cm inferior to the iliac crest in the middle third of the iliac wing. A similar advance and withdrawal technique is performed. Needle entry for the tensor fasciae latae compartment is placed 2 cm anterior and 3 cm distal to the tip of the greater trochanter. Penetration of the deep fascia should be easily felt, and additional 4 mm advancement ensures the needle is within the muscle belly.

Decompression can be performed with a posterolateral approach to the hip including a Kocher-Langenbeck or a Gibson. The Kocher-Langenbeck approach involves a curvilinear or angular incision beginning just caudal of iliac crest and lateral to PSIS, extending over the tip of the greater trochanter below along the anterolateral border of the femur. The Gibson approach differs in that the proximal portion of the incision is not directed as posteriorly and develops the interval between TFL and gluteus maximus muscles and allows for easier access to the TFL. All three gluteal compartments can be visualized and released with these approaches (Fig. 8.1). On release, evaluation of the muscle for color, contractility, consistency, and capacity to bleed should guide further debridement decisions. These approaches also allow for exploration and neuroplasty of the sciatic nerve, which should be performed in each case, especially in a patient with preoperative paresthesias or motor dysfunction in its distribution. Plans typically include additional operations for repeat inspections, debridements, and delayed closure.

Delay in diagnosis and decompression can result in permanent disability. Urgent surgical decompression can drastically improve chances for a full recovery, but

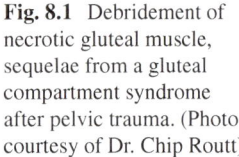

Fig. 8.1 Debridement of necrotic gluteal muscle, sequelae from a gluteal compartment syndrome after pelvic trauma. (Photo courtesy of Dr. Chip Routt)

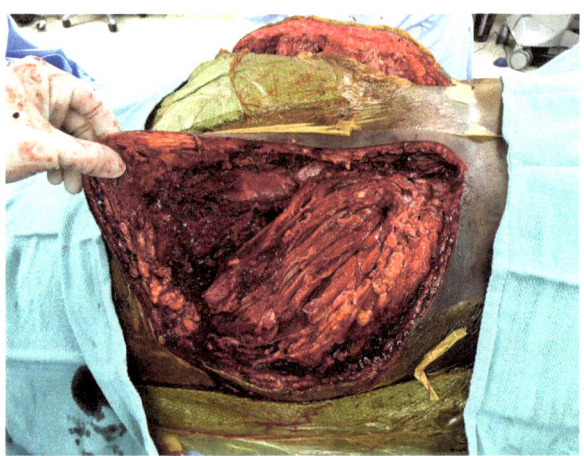

long-term outcomes include chronic hip abductor weakness with Trendelenburg gait or potentially sensory and motor changes to the foot [13]. The treatment of a missed gluteal compartment syndrome is controversial but should depend more upon the systemic condition of the patient, rather than the presence of dead musculature in the buttock. Debridement is not mandatory if the patient does not have septic myonecrosis or rhabdomyolysis and renal insufficiency.

Thigh Compartment Syndrome

Thigh compartment syndrome is typically the result of blunt trauma with motor vehicle and motorcycle collisions being the most frequent causes. In a 2010 review, they found 90% of cases attributed to blunt trauma with 44% having associated to femur fractures [15]. Other causes include gunshot wounds, arterial injuries, coagulopathies or anticoagulant therapy, burns, overexertion, reperfusion swelling, or external compression.

The thigh has three anatomical compartments: anterior, posterior, and medial. The anterior compartment includes the sartorius and quadriceps, which are all innervated by the femoral nerve. The proximal portions of the femoral artery and vein also pass through this compartment, deep to the sartorius muscle, until they pass through Hunter's canal distally. The posterior compartment includes biceps femoris, semimembranosus, semitendinosus, and the sciatic nerve. The popliteal vascular bundle passes from medial to posterior in the distal third of the thigh. The medial compartment is composed of adductors longus, magnus, and brevis as well as the gracilis muscle and the obturator neurovascular bundle.

Diagnosis of compartment syndrome in alert patients generally only needs physical examination. Physical findings are similar to other body parts including pain out of proportion, tense compartments, pain with passive stretch, and associated neurovascular changes. Muscle compartments can be tested individually with passive movements to decrease compartment volume, thereby exacerbating pain symptoms. Passive hip abduction tests the adductor compartment, knee flexion the anterior compartment, and knee extension the posterior compartment. Some surgeons may choose to use compartment pressure measurements to confirm the diagnosis in an alert patient or to make the diagnosis in an obtunded patient.

Treatment of a thigh compartment syndrome is a fasciotomy of the compartments. The anterior compartment is the most commonly affected compartment, with medial compartment involvement being more rare. The fasciotomy can be performed through a single lateral incision, allowing access for the anterior and posterior compartments. The technique for the fasciotomy involves an extensive longitudinal incision from the greater trochanter of the femur to the lateral condyle of the distal femur. The iliotibial band is incised the length of the incision, and the vastus lateralis is reflected anteriorly from the intermuscular septum releasing the anterior compartment. Incising the intermuscular septum releases the posterior compartment; however, this incision should be made away from the femur to avoid compromise of the perforating arteries traveling near the bone. The medial compartment rarely requires release once the anterior and posterior compartments have been decompressed; however, if the medial compartment remains tense, a separate anteromedial incision must be made.

A systematic review of thigh compartment syndrome revealed the majority, 59%, of thigh fasciotomy wounds were able to be closed by delayed primary closure; however, approximately 25% required skin grafting [15]. Most thigh fasciotomy wounds require multiple debridements before soft tissues are stabilized for delayed closure or split-thickness skin grafting; the average in this review was 5 days after index procedure for eventual wound closure.

Significant rates of mortality and morbidity are associated with thigh compartment syndrome. Mortality rates approach 50% due to polytraumatized or infected patients, with overall complication rates are as high as 78% in one systematic review [16]. The diagnosis also has a high association with the development of renal failure due to crush syndrome. Over half of the fasciotomy wounds in surviving patients became infected in this review. Many patients have persistent sensory deficits, motor weakness, decreased range of motion, or chronic pain of the extremity. A study examining functional outcomes found that worse results were associated with time to surgical decompression of greater than 8 hours, age over 30 years, femur fractures, high initial injury severity scores, and presence of myonecrosis at time of fasciotomy [17]. A rate as high as 40% of patients have permanent quadriceps impairment after a femur fracture, with this study finding greater than 80% with persistent thigh weakness in patients with a femur fracture and thigh ACS. The majority of patients will never recover full thigh muscle strength and have long-term functional deficits [17]. Heterotopic ossification may also be frequently visible after ACS in the thigh, although its clinical impact varies depending upon the severity and location. Decompression within 8 hours led to significantly better outcomes with strength and functional testing further giving evidence for the role of prompt fasciotomies.

Leg Compartment Syndrome

Acute compartment syndrome of the lower leg is the most frequently encountered of any area on the body. Greater than one-third of compartment syndrome cases are attributed to tibial shaft fractures [18]. It can result from both high and low-energy trauma or even atraumatic causes. Motor vehicle- and motorcycle-related injuries are the most common culprit; however, crushing injuries, burns, falls, sporting injuries, penetrating trauma, exertion, and circumferential compression can all result in ACS. Sporting events such as football and soccer have shown a strong association with development of ACS, despite being considered lower-energy trauma [19]. The rationale being that a significant local injury and inflammatory response is inflicted on younger patients with higher muscle mass who are already in a state of exertion. These injuries may not be enough to disrupt the fascial boundaries of the leg and may place them at a higher risk of an ACS. Although open fractures do not prohibit the development of a compartment syndrome, the concept of "autodecompression" is suggested by studies that report a decreased risk of ACS with high-grade open tibia fractures [18]. Regardless of the mechanism, all patients with tibial fractures should be carefully monitored with serial examinations for the potential development of an acute compartment syndrome.

The lower leg has four fascial compartments: anterior, lateral, superficial posterior, and deep posterior. The anterior compartment is very commonly involved in ACS and contains the tibialis anterior, extensor hallucis longus, extensor digitorum longus, and the deep peroneal nerve. The anterior tibial artery enters the anterior compartment through the interosseous membrane just distal to the proximal tibiofibular joint with a recurrent branch directed proximally near the tibial tubercle. The lateral compartment contains the peroneus (fibularis) longus and brevis muscles and the proximal portion of the superficial peroneal nerve, which becomes extrafascial in the middle or distal third of the leg. The superficial posterior compartment contains the medial and lateral heads of the gastrocnemius, the soleus, and plantaris muscles. The gastrocnemius muscles receive blood supply from sural branches of the popliteal artery, while the soleus is supplied by the popliteal, posterior tibial, and peroneal (fibular) arteries. The deep posterior compartment is home to the posterior tibial, flexor hallucis longus, and flexor digitorum muscles along with the posterior tibial and peroneal vessels and the tibial nerve.

Fasciotomies for ACS are often performed for all four compartments and may be done with a dual or single incision approach. The dual incision technique is most frequently used and includes anterolateral and posteromedial incisions. Regardless of the technique chosen, the anterolateral incision should be performed from the level of the proximal tibiofibular joint to the level of the distal tibiofibular joint to permit complete release and full visualization. The anterolateral incision is longitudinal and often 2–5 cm anterior to the fibular shaft or midway between the tibial crest and fibular shaft. It provides access to the anterior and lateral compartments. With the creation of subcutaneous soft tissue flaps, the intermuscular septum must be identified to ensure both compartments are released. A transverse incision may be made that allows for excellent visualization of the septum prior to longitudinal release of both of the compartments. This process is often performed in the proximal third of the leg to minimize risk of damage to the superficial peroneal nerve. The anterior compartment is released along the entire length of the compartment halfway between the septum and the tibial crest. The lateral compartment is incised posterior to the septum in line with the fibular shaft and should continue distally until the tendinous portion of the peroneal muscles is visualized. Care must be taken to protect the superficial peroneal nerve as it exits the fascia in the middle or distal third of the exposure and identification and dissection prior to anterior and lateral compartment release is recommended (see Video 8.1).

The posteromedial incision is conducted approximately 2 cm posterior to the posteromedial border of the tibia. Again the longitudinal dissection is carried out throughout the length of the leg, and the superficial posterior compartment is released initially, with exception of the lateral head of the gastrocnemius muscle. The soleal bridge, located near proximal metadiaphyseal junction of the tibia, must be completely released to adequately expose and decompress the deep posterior compartment. The deep posterior compartment is then released from the back of the tibia and is the most commonly "missed" compartment when fasciotomies are performed. The surgeon may use a Cobb elevator along the posterolateral aspect of the tibia to release this compartment and visualization of the deep posterior compartment musculature ensures it has been released (see Video 8.2).

A treatment algorithm with primary release of the anterior and lateral compartments followed by intraoperative reassessment of the superficial and deep posterior compartmental pressures has been suggested to reduce the need for four compartment releases in every case [20]. Patients presenting with compartment syndrome were initially treated with a single full-length anterolateral incision with standard release of both anterior and lateral compartments. After release, the intracompartmental pressures of both the superficial and deep posterior compartments were rechecked. Using preoperative diastolic blood pressure values, patients with ΔP values greater than 30 mmHg failed to undergo additional fasciotomies of the posterior compartments. Close postoperative observation of the patients in this study revealed no sequelae of a missed posterior compartment syndrome.

Alternatively, a single lateral incision to release all four compartments can be performed. The parafibular incision is made from the head of the fibula to the ankle, with larger subcutaneous tissue flaps created. Initial dissection is superficial to the lateral compartment, which should be followed anteriorly where the anterior intermuscular septum is identified. The anterior and lateral compartments are released similar to the anterolateral approach from the double incision technique. Next, by mobilizing the peroneal muscles anteriorly, the posterior intermuscular septum is identified which separates lateral and superficial posterior compartments. The posterior intermuscular septum joins with the transverse intermuscular septum, inserting on the posterolateral border of the fibula. Incision of these membranes and blunt elevation of the flexor hallucis longus from the posterior fibula lead to the release of the deep posterior compartment. This fascia should be completely opened and confirmed by passively moving the great toe, which can be felt in the muscle belly of the dissection. Lastly, the superficial compartment is released either by incising the posterior intermuscular septum between soleus and peroneal muscles or by retraction of a posterior subcutaneous tissue flap and direct release of the fascia covering the soleus.

Advocates for the single incision release support the decreased insult to the tenuous anteromedial skin over the tibia as well as decreased stripping of soft tissues around the tibia [21]. However, this approach is more technically challenging, and criticisms stem from concerns over adequate access to and release of the deep posterior compartment of the leg. The dual incision approach is popular due to the ease of performance and excellent exposure and is most often recommended.

A retrospective comparison of infection and nonunion rates after single versus dual incision fasciotomies did not find any statistically significant differences between the approaches, although higher numbers of infection were seen with plates versus intramedullary devices [21]. This was the first study comparing the two methods of fasciotomy for complications and was admittedly underpowered to detect potentially small differences in infection rates. In a separate investigation, Blair et al. compared groups with tibia fractures and those with tibia fractures requiring fasciotomy for acute compartment syndrome for rates of delayed union, nonunion, and infection. Their results yielded a 5-week increase in time to union, fourfold greater risk of nonunion, and fivefold greater risk of infection in tibia fractures requiring fasciotomies [22]. There are also substantial increases in the length of hospital stay and total cost associated with the need for fasciotomies to treat ACS [23]. The selection of approach may be best determined by the treating surgeon, with the goal of full release and restoration of tissue perfusion.

Wound closure is typically performed with delayed primary closure or skin graft coverage 3–7 days after fasciotomy. With the dual incision fasciotomy, priority is given to closure of the posteromedial incision due to its proximity to the tibia. Skin grafts are not aesthetically appealing and are insensate, so different methods are employed to push toward delayed primary closure. In many cases, skin grafts are inevitable, especially for the lateral wound. A vessel loop technique can be used to minimize skin retraction by interlacing the loops across the incision with staples holding at the side, gradually tensioning them to help avoid skin grafting [24]. Negative pressure wound therapy may be used for temporary coverage of fasciotomy wounds as it creates a seal decreasing contamination from hospital microorganisms, promotes wound granulation, decreases tissue edema, and improves local perfusion [25].

Foot Compartment Syndrome

Compartment syndrome of the foot is an uncommon and controversial topic. Foot compartment syndrome as a whole was underrecognized prior to the 1980s when investigation of fixed foot deformities as a result of severe foot trauma echoed similarities to Volkmann's ischemic contracture of the hand [26]. Typically, this presentation results from high-energy mechanisms such as crush injuries, motor vehicle or motorcycle collisions, or falls from height. Potential injuries vary but include isolated soft tissue trauma, forefoot fractures, Lisfranc or Chopart fracture dislocations, and calcaneal fractures. The latter, high-energy calcaneal fractures, has historically been reported to develop a foot compartment syndrome in up to 10% of cases, yet a more recent study suggests the actual incidence is lower finding only 1% of patients with an isolated calcaneal fracture underwent fasciotomy for suspected compartment syndrome [27]. Nevertheless, any patient presenting after a higher-energy mechanism, especially a crush, should be evaluated with a heightened suspicion. The development of a secondary foot compartment syndrome from more proximal injury is also described due to a communication between the deep posterior compartment of the leg and the deep central or calcaneal compartment in the foot [28].

There are considerable debate and no real consensus regarding the number of fascial compartments of the foot. Many of these studies were performed in cadavers and cannot reliably reproduce physiologic conditions [29]. At least nine compartments of the foot have been identified: three spanning the entire length of the foot (medial, lateral, and superficial), five forefoot compartments (adductor and four interossei), and a single hindfoot compartment (calcaneal) [26]. The calcaneal compartment contains the quadratus plantae muscle, lateral plantar neurovascular bundle, the posterior tibial nerve and vessels, and in some patients the medial plantar neurovascular bundle.

Diagnosis is again a combination of physical examination of the clinical presentation with an option for intracompartmental pressure monitoring. Symptoms of pain out of proportion, pain despite immobilization that is unrelieved by progressive doses of analgesics, and paresthesias are frequently seen. Signs include tense compartments and pain with passive range of motion. Passive dorsiflexion of toes decreases the volume of the interosseous compartments, thereby intensifying pain [26]. The most sensitive sensory indicators are decreased light touch and two-point discriminatory sensations, especially those with relative decreases over serial examinations [26]. Strength and pulses are poor indicators.

There is no consensus of a firm recommendation on the use of compartment measuring to the foot. This likely stems from disagreement regarding the true number of foot fascial compartments and debate about the potential of these compartments to develop pressures sufficient to cause a compartment syndrome. Continuous or even repeat monitoring of the compartments is not practical. However, it can provide further objective data helping in diagnosis. There is no firm consensus on the number of, or which, compartments that should be measured, but as the calcaneal compartment is frequently implicated as having the highest pressure readings in studies, increased attention should be paid to this compartment [28, 29]. The technique for accessing this compartment is insertion of the device 6 cm distal to the most prominent portion of the medial malleolus with insertion depth of approximately 24 mm [28]. An absolute compartment pressure >30 mmHg is generally considered an indication for emergent decompression.

The most frequently recommended approach for foot fasciotomies combines a dorsal two-incision approach with a medial plantar approach [28]. The dorsal medial incision is made just medial to the second metatarsal and allows access of the first two interosseous compartments, as well as the adductor compartment located deep to the first interosseous compartment. The dorsal lateral incision is made just lateral to the fourth metatarsal. It can be used to release the third and fourth interosseous, the lateral, and central compartments. Longitudinal dissection of the dorsal fascia is performed on both medial and lateral sides of the metatarsals with the central compartments entered after incision of the interosseous fascia. Advantages of these incisions provide exposure for fixation of midfoot trauma [29]. A separate medial plantar approach is added due to concerns of access to the calcaneal compartment from the dorsal approach [26]. This medial incision follows the length of the inferior border of the first metatarsal, a 6 cm incision beginning approximately 4 cm from the posterior border of the heel and 3 cm superior to plantar surface [26]. The abductor hallucis is retracted cranially, and the intermuscular septum is identified. Incising this septum releases the deep (calcaneal) compartment, and the quadratus plantae should bulge from the incision. Care should be taken with this step since the lateral plantar neurovascular structures are immediately deep to the septum [26]. Release of the distal tarsal tunnel through proximal extension of this medial incision may be necessary for adequate release of the calcaneal compartment [26]. Retracting this medial compartment superiorly exposes the superficial compartment, which is released longitudinally, decompressing the flexor digitorum brevis (FDB). The FDB is retracted inferiorly, and the medial fascia of the lateral compartment is visualized. Decompression of the lateral compartment is complete when the abductor digiti quinti and flexor digiti minimi are exposed [29].

Treatment with fasciotomies is not without complication, as the incisions are risks for wound infections and frequently require skin grafting. Secondary closure of wounds is typically delayed 5–7 days after fasciotomy, with skin grafting alternatively covering wounds not amenable to closure. A systematic review found that 65% of cases required skin grafts after fasciotomy [30]. Forefoot and midfoot fractures can be stabilized definitively acutely, provided primary wound closure is possible over the implants. Calcaneal fractures, however, are recommended to undergo delayed fixation 10–14 days after fasciotomy to allow swelling to decrease. Shoewear selection after soft tissue reconstruction poses another challenge that may limit long-term function. Patients commonly have residual pain and stiffness with only 10% able to return to their pre-injury state after fasciotomy [30].

There are many experienced surgeons who argue for managing the compartment syndrome conservatively, with delayed treatment of sequelae including nerve decompression, soft tissue releases, tendon transfers, osteotomies, or fusions. Although a systematic review reported that complications rates were lower for those treated with fasciotomies than those untreated, overall data comparing the two groups is lacking [30]. The treating surgeon must make the decision based upon the evaluation of the patient and their best judgment. Loss of distal perfusion should be an almost absolute indication for decompression.

An alternative approach to fasciotomies of the foot involves a "pie crusting" technique, where multiple stab incisions are made over the foot followed by blunt dissection with a hemostat [28]. The goal is to reduce pressure on the soft tissues and decrease the need for secondary soft tissue coverage; however, critics would cite the risk of inadequate release of muscular compartments.

Complications from a missed compartment syndrome include sensory alterations and the development of ischemic foot deformities. Claw toes are the most common complications, resulting from compression of the medial and lateral plantar bundles in the calcaneal compartment [28]. This ischemic insult to the quadratus plantae and interosseous muscles leads to their overpowering of these intrinsic muscles by the extrinsic muscles to the foot. Cavus foot deformities can develop as well. Neurologic complications include chronic pain, neuropathic pain, numbness, allodynia, and hyperalgesia. Ulcerations can develop secondary to the deformities, altered gait mechanics, and neuropathic changes, creating lifelong problems for some patients. Amputation is a final, but effective, treatment option in the most severe cases [28].

Summary

Compartment syndrome is a pathologic condition where intrafascial pressures increase and ultimately cause irreversible cell death if fasciotomies are not urgently performed. Diagnosis remains a challenge for all physicians and requires vigilance and frequent physical examinations. Intracompartmental measurements can be used to aid in diagnosis of obtunded patients when complete clinical examination is not possible, but measurements lack specificity and are of variable accuracy with technical errors common. Once diagnosed, urgent surgical management is simple and only requires a surgeon with anatomic knowledge and a scalpel.

References

1. Woolley SL, Smith DR. Acute compartment syndrome secondary to diabetic muscle infarction: case report and literature review. Eur J Emerg Med. 2006;13(2):113–6.
2. Garner MR, Taylor SA, Gausden E, Lyden JP. Compartment syndrome: diagnosis, management, and unique concerns in the twenty-first century. HSS J. 2014;10(2):143–52.
3. Olson SA, Glasgow RR. Acute compartment syndrome in lower extremity musculoskeletal trauma. J Am Acad Orthop Surg. 2005;13(7):436–44.
4. Whitesides TE, Heckman MM. Acute compartment syndrome: update on diagnosis and treatment. J Am Acad Orthop Surg. 1996;4(4):209–18.
5. Kortbeek JB, Al Turki SA, Ali J, Antoine JA, Bouillon B, Brasel K, et al. Advanced trauma life support, 8th edition, the evidence for change. J Trauma. 2008;64(6):1638–50.
6. Malinoski DJ, Slater MS, Mullins RJ. Crush injury and rhabdomyolysis. Crit Care Clin. 2004;20(1):171–92.

7. Kasaoka S, Todani M, Kaneko T, Kawamura Y, Oda Y, Tsuruta R, et al. Peak value of blood myoglobin predicts acute renal failure induced by rhabdomyolysis. J Crit Care. 2010;25(4): 601–4.
8. Holcomb JB, Tilley BC, Baraniuk S, Fox EE, Wade CE, Podbielski JM, et al. Transfusion of plasma, platelets, and red blood cells in a 1:1:1 vs a 1:1:2 ratio and mortality in patients with severe trauma: the PROPPR randomized clinical trial. JAMA. 2015;313(5):471–82.
9. Boody AR, Wongworawat MD. Accuracy in the measurement of compartment pressures: a comparison of three commonly used devices. J Bone Joint Surg Am. 2005;87(11): 2415–22.
10. Whitney A, O'Toole RV, Hui E, Sciadini MF, Pollak AN, Manson TT, et al. Do one-time intracompartmental pressure measurements have a high false-positive rate in diagnosing compartment syndrome? J Trauma Acute Care Surg. 2014;76(2):479–83.
11. McQueen MM, Court-Brown CM. Compartment monitoring in tibial fractures. The pressure threshold for decompression. J Bone Joint Surg Br. 1996;78(1):99–104.
12. Large TM, Agel J, Holtzman DJ, Benirschke SK, Krieg JC. Interobserver variability in the measurement of lower leg compartment pressures. J Orthop Trauma. 2015;29(7): 316–21.
13. Henson JT, Roberts CS, Giannoudis PV. Gluteal compartment syndrome. Acta Orthop Belg. 2009;75(2):147–52.
14. David V, Thambiah J, Kagda FH, Kumar VP. Bilateral gluteal compartment syndrome. A case report. J Bone Joint Surg Am. 2005;87(11):2541–5.
15. Ojike NI, Roberts CS, Giannoudis PV. Compartment syndrome of the thigh: a systematic review. Injury. 2010;41(2):133–6.
16. Schwartz JT Jr, Brumback RJ, Lakatos R, Poka A, Bathon GH, Burgess AR. Acute compartment syndrome of the thigh. A spectrum of injury. J Bone Joint Surg Am. 1989;71(3): 392–400.
17. Mithoefer K, Lhowe DW, Vrahas MS, Altman DT, Erens V, Altman GT. Functional outcome after acute compartment syndrome of the thigh. J Bone Joint Surg Am. 2006;88(4): 729–37.
18. McQueen MM, Gaston P, Court-Brown CM. Acute compartment syndrome. Who is at risk? J Bone Joint Surg Br. 2000;82(2):200–3.
19. Wind TC, Saunders SM, Barfield WR, Mooney JF 3rd, Hartsock LA. Compartment syndrome after low-energy tibia fractures sustained during athletic competition. J Orthop Trauma. 2012;26(1):33–6.
20. Tornetta P 3rd, Puskas BL, Wang K. Compartment syndrome of the leg associated with fracture: an algorithm to avoid releasing the posterior compartments. J Orthop Trauma. 2016;30(7):381–6.
21. Bible JE, McClure DJ, Mir HR. Analysis of single-incision versus dual-incision fasciotomy for tibial fractures with acute compartment syndrome. J Orthop Trauma. 2013;27(11): 607–11.
22. Blair JA, Stoops TK, Doarn MC, Kemper D, Erdogan M, Griffing R, et al. Infection and nonunion after fasciotomy for compartment syndrome associated with tibia fractures: a matched cohort comparison. J Orthop Trauma. 2016;30(7):392–6.
23. Crespo AM, Manoli A 3rd, Konda SR, Egol KA. Development of compartment syndrome negatively impacts length of stay and cost after tibia fracture. J Orthop Trauma. 2015;29(7): 312–5.
24. Asgari MM, Spinelli HM. The vessel loop shoelace technique for closure of fasciotomy wounds. Ann Plast Surg. 2000;44(2):225–9.
25. Kanakaris NK, Thanasas C, Keramaris N, Kontakis G, Granick MS, Giannoudis PV. The efficacy of negative pressure wound therapy in the management of lower extremity trauma: review of clinical evidence. Injury. 2007;38(Suppl 5):S9–18.
26. Fulkerson E, Razi A, Tejwani N. Review: acute compartment syndrome of the foot. Foot Ankle Int. 2003;24(2):180–7.

27. Thakur NA, McDonnell M, Got CJ, Arcand N, Spratt KF, DiGiovanni CW. Injury patterns causing isolated foot compartment syndrome. J Bone Joint Surg Am. 2012;94(11):1030–5.
28. Dodd A, Le I. Foot compartment syndrome: diagnosis and management. J Am Acad Orthop Surg. 2013;21(11):657–64.
29. Frink M, Hildebrand F, Krettek C, Brand J, Hankemeier S. Compartment syndrome of the lower leg and foot. Clin Orthop Relat Res. 2010;468(4):940–50.
30. Ojike NI, Roberts CS, Giannoudis PV. Foot compartment syndrome: a systematic review of the literature. Acta Orthop Belg. 2009;75(5):573–80.

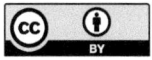

Chapter 9
Fasciotomy Wound Management

Vasilios G. Igoumenou, Zinon T. Kokkalis, and Andreas F. Mavrogenis

Problem Background

- Surgical fasciotomy is the only effective treatment, offering an immediate decrease in the compartment pressure and an increase in the volume of the affected muscle compartment through the release of the skin and muscle fascia.
- Complications of fasciotomy include long hospital stay, wound infection and osteomyelitis, need for further surgery for delayed wound closure or skin grafting, scarring, delayed bone healing, pain and nerve injury, permanent muscle weakness, chronic venous insufficiency, cosmetic problems, and an overall increased cost of care.
- However, closure of fasciotomy wounds is challenging, and a plethora of techniques have been proposed.
- With no consensus existing in the literature regarding the best method for closure of fasciotomy wounds, the technique applied each time is based mostly on surgeon's preference and other variables, such as the condition of the tissues surrounding the wound, availability of materials and devices, patients' environment and preference, and institutional financial resources.

The original version of this chapter was revised. The correction to this chapter can be found at https://doi.org/10.1007/978-3-030-22331-1_18

V. G. Igoumenou · A. F. Mavrogenis (✉)
First Department of Orthopedics, National and Kapodistrian University of Athens, School of Medicine, Athens, Attica, Greece
e-mail: afm@otenet.gr

Z. T. Kokkalis
Department of Orthopedics, University of Patras, Patras, Achaia, Greece

© The Author(s) 2019
C. Mauffrey et al. (eds.), *Compartment Syndrome*,
https://doi.org/10.1007/978-3-030-22331-1_9

Introduction

Acute compartment syndrome is a surgical emergency, in the setting of which immediate actions should be taken to avert muscle and nerve cell death [1, 2]. In order to prevent irreversible tissue necrosis, treatment aims to restore muscle perfusion as quickly as possible [1, 3]. Surgical fasciotomy presents the only effective treatment, offering an immediate decrease in the compartment pressure and an increase in the volume of the affected muscle compartment through the release of the skin and muscle fascia [1, 3]. Nonetheless, fasciotomy carries its own risks and complications, including long hospital stay, wound infection and osteomyelitis, need for further surgery for delayed wound closure or skin grafting, scarring, delayed bone healing, pain and nerve injury, permanent muscle weakness, chronic venous insufficiency, cosmetic problems, and an overall increased cost of care (Fig. 9.1) [2–5].

To reduce the risk of complications, the fasciotomy wound should be closed as quickly as possible [6]. However, early primary wound closure is not recommended as it may lead to increased muscle pressure and recurrent compartment syndrome [2, 5, 7, 8]. As a result, closure of fasciotomy wounds is challenging, and a plethora of techniques have been proposed. With no consensus existing in the literature regarding the best method for closure of fasciotomy wounds, the technique applied each time is based mostly on surgeon's preference and other variables, such as the condition of the tissues surrounding the wound, availability of materials and devices, patients' environment and preference, and institutional financial resources [7, 9]. This chapter aims to summarize the available techniques employed in fasciotomy wound closure and to discuss the indications, advantages, disadvantages, and complications of these techniques in a way that readers may find useful and educative.

Fig. 9.1 (**a**) A 42-year-old man with a crush injury of the leg with tibia and fibula fracture. (**b**) Fasciotomy was done, but because of muscle necrosis and sepsis, he ended with a knee disarticulation

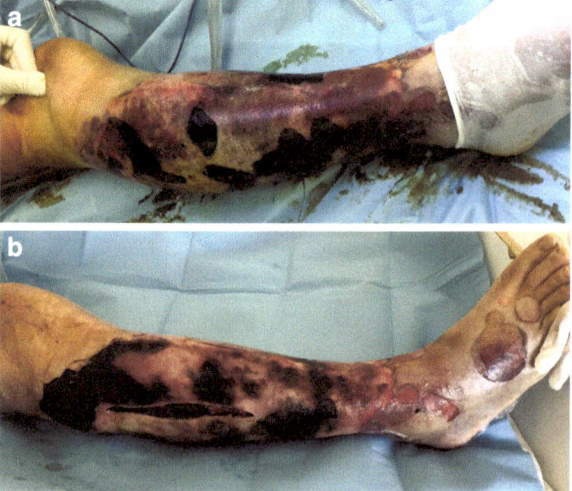

Early Primary Wound Closure

Early primary wound closure of fasciotomy wounds, apart from being rarely possible due to edematous tissues, is also not recommended since it may lead to recurrent compartment syndrome [7]. Split-thickness skin grafting has been widely used for fasciotomy wound closure, as it has been thought to reduce patient morbidity from wound complications and delayed rehabilitation compared to immediately primarily or secondarily closed fasciotomy wounds [10, 11]. The use of skin grafts is associated with donor site morbidity, infection, lack of sensation over the fasciotomy site, risk of graft nonadherence, and poor cosmesis that, at times, requires scar revision or resection [6, 7, 9, 12, 13]. Yet, split-thickness skin grafting remains a viable option when other closure techniques fail or in special cases, as in persistently dehiscent wounds, in burnt or friable wound edges, and in very large skin defects [1, 7, 9]. Additionally, split-thickness skin grafting represents frequently a benchmark for evaluating complications, safety, efficacy, and cost-effectiveness of other newly introduced closure techniques [7, 12].

Delayed Primary Wound Closure

After fasciotomy, the wound is usually managed open and dressed sterilely with moist dressings to protect the tissue from drying and retraction [2, 5]. Alternatively, negative pressure wound therapy (NPWT) can be employed [2, 5, 7, 9, 13–20], or numerous techniques can be performed for staged wound closure aiming for gradual approximation of skin edges once the edema begins to resolve (Table 9.1) [7, 21–51].

Table 9.1 Summary of published studies on dynamic dermatotraction and static tension devices for fasciotomy wound closure

Study	Level of evidence	Technique	Description
Dynamic dermatotraction mechanical devices			
Bulstrode et al. [46][a]	IV	*Op Site closure technique*	Adhesive film dressing (Op Site) applied across the fasciotomy wound is reduced gradually by means of a tensioning rod stuck to the center of the dressing
Hirshowitz et al. [39][a]	IV	*U-shaped hooked arms*	Two pins are threaded through the dermis of the wound margins, and two U-shaped hooked arms engage the pins through the overlying skin surface. A threaded screw passes through the centers of the arms, and when the screw is turned by a tension knob at its free end, the distal arm, which is loose, rides over the screw and is pulled over, facilitating reapproximation

(continued)

Table 9.1 (continued)

Study	Level of evidence	Technique	Description
Narayanan et al. [34]	IV	*Sure-closure* (Life Medical Sciences, Princeton, NJ)	Modification of U-shaped arms. The device is tightened in cycles; 30–90 minutes of tightening are interrupted by 10-minute periods of loosening ("load cycling"). The fasciotomy wound can be even closed intraoperatively
Caruso et al. [47]	IV		
Hussman et al. [35]	IV		
McKeneey et al. [40]	IV	*STAR* (suture tension adjustment reel; WoundTEK Inc., Newport, RI)	One anchoring and one winding shell are connected by heavy-duty nylon mattress suture. The winder shell is tightened at the bedside with the use of a wrench, reapproximating the wound edges, and the wounds are closed under local anesthesia over several days
Wiger et al. [44]	IV	*External tissue extension* (ETE, Hojmed, Loddekopinge, Sweden)	Dermal traction is achieved by silicone bands passing through a slot in a plastic unit consisting of a needle and two friction stoppers counted on a silicone string
Bjarnesen et al. [48]	IV		
Janzing et al. [49]	III	*Marburger plates* (described by Hessmann)	Plates placed along the sides of the wound joined by sutures and progressively tightened
Taylor et al. [50]	IV	*Dynamic wound closure device* (DWC; Canica, Almonte, Ontario, Canada)	Cleated or adhesive skin anchors laced together with silicone elastomers, which can be individually tightened, allowing for constant tension over the entire wound
Singh et al. [42]	IV		
Barnea et al. [38]	IV	*Wisebands* wound closure device (Wisebands Company Ltd, Misgav, Israel)	A tension feedback control device measures the tension on the wound edges during tightening and adjusts accordingly to maintain an appropriate level of tension
Medina et al. [41]	III	*Silver bullet wound closure device* (SBWCD; Boehringer Laboratories, Norristown, PA)	A 9.5-cm stainless steel instrument resembling a silver bullet is sutured into the middle of the wound and tightened daily through the rotation of an internal cylinder gradually contracting the wound
Manista et al. [51]	IV	*DermaClose RC* (Wound Care Technologies, Inc., Chanhassen, MN)	Continuous external tissue expander, providing a constant traction force on surrounding wound skin edge. Barbed skin anchors are stapled uniformly around the wound and a tensiomer applies a continuous controlled pulling force on a heavy suture that is "laced" to the skin anchors

Table 9.1 (continued)

Study	Level of evidence	Technique	Description
Topaz et al. [43]	IV	*TopClosure* 3S system (IVT Medical Ltd., Ra'anana, Israel)	Comprises two attachment plates that are interconnected by a long, flexible approximation strap. The strap links the opposing plates, enabling approximation and advancing the plates by incremental pull on the strap. The plates are attached to the skin either by staples/sutures or by hypoallergenic, biocompatible adhesive
Static tension devices			
Mbubaegbu and Stallard [33][a]	V	*Plaster strips*	Serially applied longitudinal plaster strips on either side of the wound bridged by plaster bridging strips, and twice weekly the strips are changed, so as to gradually achieve wound closure
Harrah [32]	IV	*Steri-Strips* (3M Surgical Products, St Paul, MN)	Steri-Strips are used instead of plaster
Rogers [12][a]	III	*Staged linear closure*	Progressive wound closure as the swelling subsides. Areas left open between stages are covered with a vacuum-assisted wound dressing

[a]Original report of the technique

Negative Pressure Wound Therapy

Negative pressure wound therapy (NPWT) or vacuum-assisted wound closure can be applied in various ways in fasciotomy wound management depending on different wound conditions, progress of healing, and surgeon's preference. First, it can be used as an alternative to the wet-dry dressings, which are traditionally used immediately after fasciotomy [5, 7]. Second, NPWT can be used as a definite treatment of fasciotomy wounds until wound healing is accomplished [1, 2, 5–7, 9, 13]. Third, NPWT can be used as an adjunct to other closure techniques [2, 7, 9, 13]. Initially introduced in the late 1990s [14], NPWT has been widely used in the management of challenging wounds. It involves the use of a foam dressing, covered by an adhesive drape that is connected to a vacuum pump in order to create subatmospheric pressure on the wound that is equally distributed, creating a controlled closed wound [9, 14]. Its therapeutic properties regarding fasciotomy wounds result from the positive effects of subatmospheric pressure. Moreover, as excess fluid is drained from the affected compartment, extracellular edema and tissue swelling are reduced, thereby compartment pressure is further decreased [1, 5, 7, 9, 13, 15]. Furthermore, local blood flow is improved, a moist environment is preserved, retraction of wound edges is prevented, bacterial count may also be decreased, and angiogenesis can be stimulated, leading ideally to improved wound healing and decreased risk of infection [1, 5, 7, 9, 13–15]. Researchers have found that with NPWT fasciotomy wounds can be closed earlier and with less need for skin grafting; when used as a bolster for skin grafts, it has been found to promote graft adherence and prevent potential hematoma or seroma formation [13, 16, 17].

The drawbacks of NWPT compared to other closure techniques in terms of morbidity, cost-effectiveness, and length of treatment have been reported in related studies [6, 7, 15, 18]. More specifically, in a recent randomized trial, NWPT was associated with increased need for skin grafting, increased cost, and longer duration of treatment as compared to the shoelace technique [6]. Increased need for skin grafting after NPWT was also found in another large retrospective study compared to patients treated with saline-soaked gauze packing and vessel loop dermatotraction [18], which is in accordance with the findings from other studies in which NPWT was related to incomplete healing and increased need for additional skin grafts, thereby increasing duration and cost of treatment [7, 15]. NPWT has been further associated with overgranulation that may delay epithelialization and with granulation tissue growing into the sponge creating nidi prone to inflammation or infection [6, 19]. In cases with massive muscle swelling, the wound edges cannot be sufficiently contracted by NPWT, and the tissues tend to become increasingly rigid due to granulation, further limiting complete approximation of the skin margins [6]. The use of NPWT in wounds with active bleeding should be avoided as well, since arterial erosion and bleeding have been reported [20]. In the same scenario, when a vascular reconstruction has been performed, NPWT is contraindicated [7].

Gradual Suture Approximation

Cohn et al. [21] were the first to describe a gradual suture approximation technique for fasciotomy wounds named the shoelace technique that represents one of the most widely applied methods in the management of fasciotomy wounds. Staples are placed along the wound edges, and a vessel loop is threaded through these staples in a crisscross fashion, like a shoelace (Fig. 9.2). Afterward, the loop is tied under light tension and tightened every 48 hours at the bedside [21]. When the wound edges are adequately approximated for suturing (typically within 1 cm), a second operation is performed and delayed primary closure can be accomplished [13, 22].

The shoelace technique is a simple, safe, and inexpensive method to bring the skin margins together gradually as swelling resolves [7, 13]. It does not interfere with external fixators or limb and patient mobilization and usually results in a fine linear scar, without the need for skin grafting [7, 23]. Although not being a major

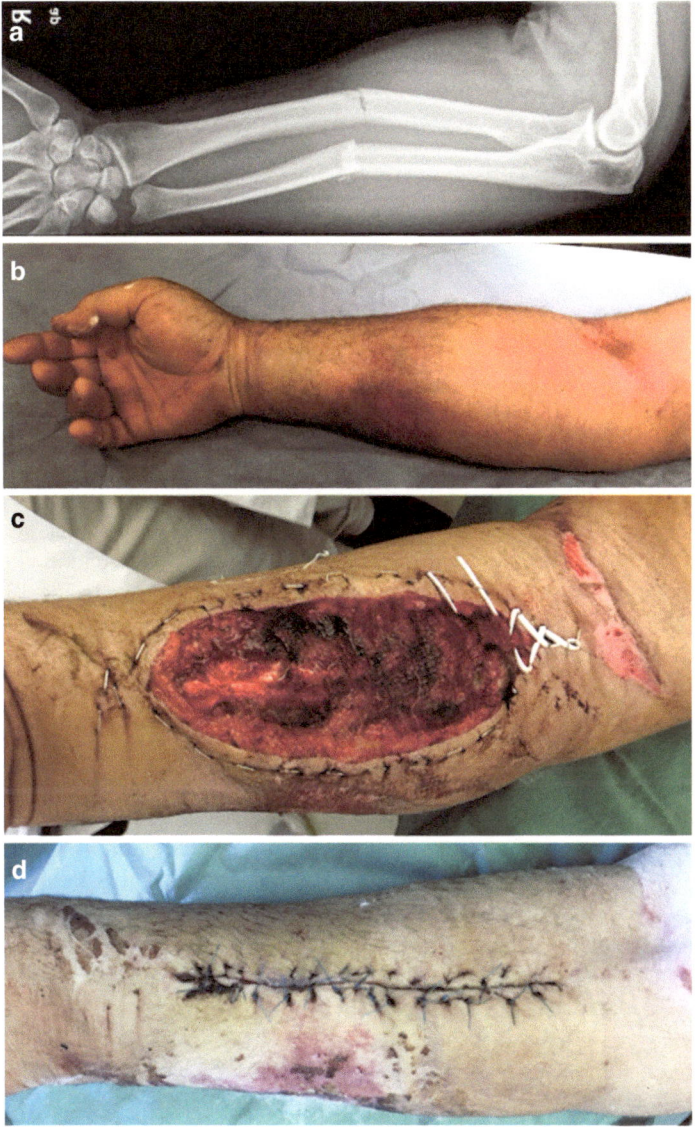

Fig. 9.2 (a) A 46-year-old man with a two-bone forearm fracture. (b) Clinical examination at presentation showed severe, constant pain, increased pain on passive stretch of the wrist and fingers, paresthesias, and weakness at the distribution of the median and ulnar nerves; radial artery pulses were intact. Fracture osteosynthesis and (c) volar fasciotomy was done with gradual fasciotomy wound approximation with a shoelace technique. (d) Delayed primary fasciotomy wound closure was done at 2 weeks, (e) with excellent cosmesis and function at 6 months postoperatively

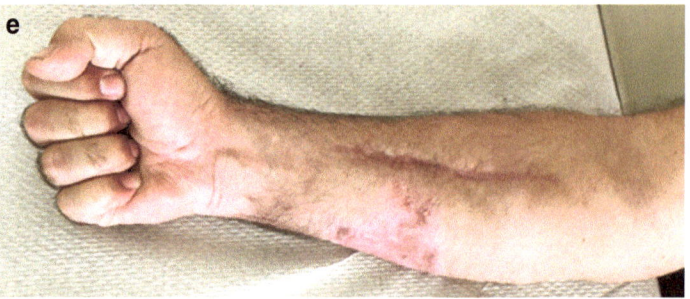

Fig. 9.2 (continued)

drawback, staple detachment often occurs secondary to point loading from tightening or limb mobilization; therefore, staples need to be checked and replaced where necessary. Marginal ischemia and/or skin necrosis may rarely occur, again due to point loading at the staple sites [7]. Several modifications of the original technique have been described, aiming to improve the technique and eliminate its weaknesses. Nylon sutures have been used instead of vessel loops, as the latter are not designed for wound closure and lack the essential strength to close large defects [7, 24]. The use of paper clip to secure the vessel loop ends was also described as an alternative to knots, in order to maintain tension [23]. The use of subcutaneous [25] or intracutaneous nylon sutures [22, 26] that are gradually tightened at bedside may achieve direct final closure of the wound without the need for a reoperation. However, replacing these sutures in case they break during approximation is not as easy as replacing sutures or loops threaded through staples [7, 25]. Furthermore, they present an increased risk for skin necrosis. A modification of these techniques is to pass the sutures through catheters, to avoid direct contact of the sutures with the underlying soft tissues [27]. Gradual tightening of a silicon sheet that is fixed without tension and covers completely the wound has been proposed as a safe, painless and cost-effective method that may be associated with a reduced risk of infection and improved cosmetic results [28]. Other surgeons described the application of Ty-Raps (Thomas & Betts, Memphis, Tennessee, USA) that are stapled to the skin and individually tightened each day [29].

Callanan and Macey used fine subcuticular Kirschner wires along both sides of fasciotomy wounds with an elastic band that was stapled in a shoelace pattern to the wound edges and, at the same time, to the underlying Kirschner wires, thus creating an even distribution of tension along the skin edges during approximation, thereby preventing ischemia [30]. A simpler suture technique described by Dahners for fasciotomy wounds is the running "near-near-far-far" stitch; the near stitch is passed 5 mm to 10 mm from the wound edge, and the far stitch is passed 3 cm to 6 cm from the wound edge [31]. According to Dahners, running of the suture balances the tension throughout the wound and allows the suture to be tightened once swelling has receded [31].

In general, suture approximation techniques are widely popular in the management of fasciotomy wounds because of good to excellent outcomes with high wound closure rates, use of inexpensive and easily accessible materials that are available in healthcare facilities with limited resources, and ease of application and the suture tightening that can be safely performed even in an outpatient setting [7, 9, 29]. Wound closure with suture approximation is expected to occur within 5 days to 3 weeks [6, 7, 22, 23]. Complications such as ischemia or increase of compartmental pressures, though rare, may occur; therefore, continuous evaluation of the wound is recommended.

Dynamic Dermatotraction and Static Tension Devices

Although numerous methods and devices have been developed for the management of fasciotomy wounds, none managed to gain wide popularity, while their use has been mainly reported as single specific-center experience [7]. Static and dynamic traction techniques have been described with variable results, effectiveness, and related complications. Regarding the application of static tension methods [12, 32, 33], plaster and Steri-Strips cannot reliably apply forces required to close large fasciotomy wounds with severely protruding muscles [7]. Staged linear closure, on the other hand, requires multiple operative procedures until wound closure is achieved; NPWT should be additionally applied in staged linear fasciotomy wound closure, as originally described by Rogers et al. [12], therefore further increasing the cost of treatment. Dynamic dermatotraction mechanical devices have yet to prove their effectiveness and simplicity, since they are associated with significant costs without decreasing morbidity as compared to other techniques [9]. The sure-closure technique as described by Narayanan [34] was reported to achieve primary wound closure; intraoperative wound closure was obtained in 21 of 24 patients in a maximum of 100 minutes. The technique relies on skin's viscoelastic properties; periods of skin tightening (30–90 minutes) are interchanged ("load cycling") with short periods (10 minutes) of loosening. However, apart from being expensive, when used for long periods of time, it may increase intracompartmental pressures and thereby the potential for skin and muscle necrosis [35].

Higher-level studies evaluating and comparing techniques for static and dynamic delayed fasciotomy wound healing are yet to be reported [36]. These techniques exploit skin's inherent viscoelastic properties. Mechanical creep defined as the elongation of the skin with a constant load over time beyond intrinsic extensibility is the main property of the skin on which all dermatotraction techniques rely [7, 37]. However, regardless of the device or method applied, the surgeons should always refer to the basic principles of tissue (skin) expansion, with the most important being that application of any tension must be deferred until the edema of the injured limb subsides. In case skin expansion is initiated too early and/or too rapidly, the risk for skin edges necrosis, delayed healing, recurrent compartment syndrome, infection, failure of wound closure, and hypertrophic scarring is increased [11, 22, 34, 35, 38–44]. Signs of excessive tension are patient discomfort during or after manipulations and the pale color of skin ischemia [7].

Secondary Wound Closure

It is generally accepted for fasciotomy wounds to be initially left open and then managed by delayed primary closure. However, in the past, fasciotomy wounds were managed open, and closure was attempted by secondary intention [7, 9]. This technique has been abandoned nonetheless, due to unacceptable high infection rates, increased risk of muscle necrosis and sepsis, prolonged hospitalization, delay in rehabilitation, and excessive scarring [7, 9, 11, 45]. It may be reserved though only for fasciotomy wounds, where delayed primary closure has failed due to underlying infection or wound dehiscence [7].

Conclusion

Currently, there is no consensus regarding the optimal technique for fasciotomy wound closure. High-level studies are missing, and the use of complex devices for wound closure after fasciotomy is not substantially advantageous over standard techniques such as suture approximation techniques [7, 9, 13]. Primary wound closure with direct wound edge approximation should be avoided due to high risk of tissue necrosis and persistent or recurrent compartment syndrome. After the initial management, fasciotomy wounds should be regularly inspected as surgical debridement may be necessary within 48–72 hours [2] until the wound presents viable, non-necrotic tissues and muscles [5, 13]. For patients with poor compliance, atrophic or friable skin, infection, or questionable viability of the skin and surrounding tissues, skin grafting is probably the most preferable option. The advantage of NPWT and dermatotraction mechanical devices over shoelace and simple suture techniques has not been documented [6, 7, 9]. In terms of complications though, NPWT has been associated with the lowest rates (2.49%), followed by suture approximation (14.83%) and dynamic dermatotraction (18.4%). It is therefore implied that for patients at high risk of complications, NPWT may be the treatment of choice, whereas when primary closure is the main goal, suture approximation or dynamic dermatotraction devices should be preferred [9]. Treating surgeons should be familiar with every technique, as well as with their advantages and limitations, and patients' selection should be performed for the optimum functional and aesthetic outcomes.

References

1. McLaughlin N, Heard H, Kelham S. Acute and chronic compartment syndromes: know when to act fast. JAAPA. 2014;27(6):23–6. https://doi.org/10.1097/01.JAA.0000446999.10176.13.
2. von Keudell AG, Weaver MJ, Appleton PT, Bae DS, Dyer GSM, Heng M, Jupiter JB, Vrahas MS. Diagnosis and treatment of acute extremity compartment syndrome. Lancet. 2015;386(10000):1299–310. https://doi.org/10.1016/S0140-6736(15)00277-9.

3. Schmidt AH. Acute compartment syndrome. Injury. 2017;48(Suppl 1):S22–5. https://doi.org/10.1016/j.injury.2017.04.024.
4. Reverte MM, Dimitriou R, Kanakaris NK, Giannoudis PV. What is the effect of compartment syndrome and fasciotomies on fracture healing in tibial fractures? Injury. 2011;42(12):1402–7. https://doi.org/10.1016/j.injury.2011.09.007.
5. Schmidt AH. Acute compartment syndrome. Orthop Clin North Am. 2016;47(3):517–25. https://doi.org/10.1016/j.ocl.2016.02.001.
6. Kakagia D, Karadimas EJ, Drosos G, Ververidis A, Trypsiannis G, Verettas D. Wound closure of leg fasciotomy: comparison of vacuum-assisted closure versus shoelace technique. A randomised study. Injury. 2014;45(5):890–3. https://doi.org/10.1016/j.injury.2012.02.002.
7. Kakagia D. How to close a limb fasciotomy wound: an overview of current techniques. Int J Low Extrem Wounds. 2015;14(3):268–76. https://doi.org/10.1177/1534734614550310.
8. Olson SA, Glasgow RR. Acute compartment syndrome in lower extremity musculoskeletal trauma. J Am Acad Orthop Surg. 2005;13(7):436–44.
9. Jauregui JJ, Yarmis SJ, Tsai J, Onuoha KO, Illical E, Paulino CB. Fasciotomy closure techniques. J Orthop Surg (Hong Kong). 2017;25(1):2309499016684724. https://doi.org/10.1177/2309499016684724.
10. Bibi C, Nyska M, Howard C, Dekel S. Compartmental syndrome due to high velocity missile injury of the calf: use of immediate mesh skin grafting. Mil Med. 1991;156(8):436–8.
11. Johnson SB, Weaver FA, Yellin AE, Kelly R, Bauer M. Clinical results of decompressive dermotomy-fasciotomy. Am J Surg. 1992;164(3):286–90.
12. Rogers GF, Maclellan RA, Liu AS, Taghinia AH, Labow BI, Meara JG, Greene AK. Extremity fasciotomy wound closure: comparison of skin grafting to staged linear closure. J Plast Reconstr Aesthet Surg. 2013;66(3):e90–1. https://doi.org/10.1016/j.bjps.2012.11.014.
13. Shadgan B, Menon M, Sanders D, Berry G, Martin C Jr, Duffy P, Stephen D, O'Brien PJ. Current thinking about acute compartment syndrome of the lower extremity. Can J Surg. 2010;53(5):329–34.
14. Argenta LC, Morykwas MJ. Vacuum-assisted closure: a new method for wound control and treatment: clinical experience. Ann Plast Surg. 1997;38(6):563–76; discussion 577.
15. Zannis J, Angobaldo J, Marks M, DeFranzo A, David L, Molnar J, Argenta L. Comparison of fasciotomy wound closures using traditional dressing changes and the vacuum-assisted closure device. Ann Plast Surg. 2009;62(4):407–9. https://doi.org/10.1097/SAP.0b013e3181881b29.
16. Blackburn JH 2nd, Boemi L, Hall WW, Jeffords K, Hauck RM, Banducci DR, Graham WP 3rd. Negative-pressure dressings as a bolster for skin grafts. Ann Plast Surg. 1998;40(5):453–7.
17. Yang CC, Chang DS, Webb LX. Vacuum-assisted closure for fasciotomy wounds following compartment syndrome of the leg. J Surg Orthop Adv. 2006;15(1):19–23.
18. Matt SE, Johnson LS, Shupp JW, Kheirbek T, Sava JA. Management of fasciotomy wounds-- does the dressing matter? Am Surg. 2011;77(12):1656–60.
19. Saeed MU, Kennedy DJ. A retained sponge is a complication of vacuum-assisted closure therapy. Int J Low Extrem Wounds. 2007;6(3):153–4. https://doi.org/10.1177/1534734607305597.
20. White RA, Miki RA, Kazmier P, Anglen JO. Vacuum-assisted closure complicated by erosion and hemorrhage of the anterior tibial artery. J Orthop Trauma. 2005;19(1):56–9.
21. Cohn BT, Shall J, Berkowitz M. Forearm fasciotomy for acute compartment syndrome: a new technique for delayed primary closure. Orthopedics. 1986;9(9):1243–6.
22. Janzing HM, Broos PL. Dermatotraction: an effective technique for the closure of fasciotomy wounds: a preliminary report of fifteen patients. J Orthop Trauma. 2001;15(6):438–41.
23. Sawant MR, Hallett JP. The paper-clip modification to the vessel loop 'shoelace' technique for delayed primary closure of fasciotomies. Injury. 2001;32(8):619–20.
24. Almekinders LC. Tips of the trade #32. Gradual closure of fasciotomy wounds. Orthop Rev. 1991;20(1):82–4.
25. Chiverton N, Redden JF. A new technique for delayed primary closure of fasciotomy wounds. Injury. 2000;31(1):21–4.

26. Riedl S, Werner J, Gohring U, Meeder PJ. The pre-positioned intracutaneous suture--a method for treatment of soft tissue defects after fascia splitting in acute compartment syndrome. Chirurg. 1994;65(11):1052–5.

27. Galois L, Pauchot J, Pfeffer F, Kermarrec I, Traversari R, Mainard D, Delagoutte JP. Modified shoelace technique for delayed primary closure of the thigh after acute compartment syndrome. Acta Orthop Belg. 2002;68(1):63–7.

28. Walker T, Gruler M, Ziemer G, Bail DH. The use of a silicon sheet for gradual wound closure after fasciotomy. J Vasc Surg. 2012;55(6):1826–8. https://doi.org/10.1016/j.jvs.2011.12.009.

29. Govaert GA, van Helden S. Ty-raps in trauma: a novel closing technique of extremity fasciotomy wounds. J Trauma. 2010;69(4):972–5. https://doi.org/10.1097/TA.0b013e3181f2d9d3.

30. Callanan I, Macey A. Closure of fasciotomy wounds. A technical modification. J Hand Surg Br. 1997;22(2):264–5.

31. Dahners LE. The running near-near-far-far stitch for closure of fasciotomies and other large wounds. Orthopedics. 2003;26(4):383–4.

32. Harrah J, Gates R, Carl J, Harrah JD. A simpler, less expensive technique for delayed primary closure of fasciotomies. Am J Surg. 2000;180(1):55–7.

33. Mbubaegbu CE, Stallard MC. A method of fasciotomy wound closure. Injury. 1996;27(9):613–5.

34. Narayanan K, Futrell JW, Bentz M, Hurwitz D. Comparative clinical study of the sure-closure device with conventional wound closure techniques. Ann Plast Surg. 1995;35(5):485–91.

35. Hussmann J, Kucan JO, Zamboni WA. Elevated compartmental pressures after closure of a forearm burn wound with a skin-stretching device. Burns. 1997;23(2):154–6.

36. Arain AR, Cole K, Sullivan C, Banerjee S, Kazley J, Uhl RL. Tissue expanders with a focus on extremity reconstruction. Expert Rev Med Devices. 2018;15(2):145–55. https://doi.org/10.1080/17434440.2018.1426457.

37. Wilhelmi BJ, Blackwell SJ, Mancoll JS, Phillips LG. Creep vs. stretch: a review of the viscoelastic properties of skin. Ann Plast Surg. 1998;41(2):215–9.

38. Barnea Y, Gur E, Amir A, Leshem D, Zaretski A, Miller E, Shafir R, Weiss J. Delayed primary closure of fasciotomy wounds with Wisebands, a skin- and soft tissue-stretch device. Injury. 2006;37(6):561–6. https://doi.org/10.1016/j.injury.2006.02.056.

39. Hirshowitz B, Lindenbaum E, Har-Shai Y. A skin-stretching device for the harnessing of the viscoelastic properties of skin. Plast Reconstr Surg. 1993;92(2):260–70.

40. McKenney MG, Nir I, Fee T, Martin L, Lentz K. A simple device for closure of fasciotomy wounds. Am J Surg. 1996;172(3):275–7. https://doi.org/10.1016/S0002-9610(96)00107-9.

41. Medina C, Spears J, Mitra A. The use of an innovative device for wound closure after upper extremity fasciotomy. Hand (N Y). 2008;3(2):146–51. https://doi.org/10.1007/s11552-007-9082-y.

42. Singh N, Bluman E, Starnes B, Andersen C. Dynamic wound closure for decompressive leg fasciotomy wounds. Am Surg. 2008;74(3):217–20.

43. Topaz M, Carmel NN, Silberman A, Li MS, Li YZ. The TopClosure(R) 3S System, for skin stretching and a secure wound closure. Eur J Plast Surg. 2012;35(7):533–43. https://doi.org/10.1007/s00238-011-0671-1.

44. Wiger P, Blomqvist G, Styf J. Wound closure by dermatotraction after fasciotomy for acute compartment syndrome. Scand J Plast Reconstr Surg Hand Surg. 2000;34(4):315–20.

45. Jensen SL, Sandermann J. Compartment syndrome and fasciotomy in vascular surgery. A review of 57 cases. Eur J Vasc Endovasc Surg. 1997;13(1):48–53.

46. Bulstrode CJ, King JB, Worpole R, Ham RJ. A simple method for closing fasciotomies. Ann R Coll Surg Engl. 1985;67(2):119–20.

47. Caruso DM, King TJ, Tsujimura RB, Weiland DE, Schiller WR. Primary closure of fasciotomy incisions with a skin-stretching device in patients with burn and trauma. J Burn Care Rehabil. 1997;18(2):125–32.

48. Bjarnesen JP, Wester JU, Siemssen SS, Blomqvist G, Jensen NK. External tissue stretching for closing skin defects in 22 patients. Acta Orthop Scand. 1996;67(2):182–4.

49. Janzing HMJ, Broos PLO. Dermatotraction: an effective technique for the closure of fasci-otomy wounds: a preliminary report of fifteen patients. J Orthop Trauma. 2001;6:438–41.
50. Taylor RC, Reitsma BJ, Sarazin S, Bell MG. Early results using a dynamic method for delayed primary closure of fasciotomy wounds. J Am Coll Surg. 2003;197:872–8.
51. Manista GC, Dennis A, Kaminsky M. Surgical management of compartment syndrome and the gradual closure of a fasciotomy wound using a DermaClose device. Trauma Case Rep. 2018;14:1–4.

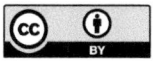

Chapter 10
Foot Compartment Syndrome Controversy

**Julian G. Lugo-Pico, Amiethab Aiyer, Jonathan Kaplan,
and Anish R. Kadakia**

Background

- Foot compartment syndrome is a rare but debilitating condition.
- Clinical presentation and evaluation can differ with classically reported signs and symptoms of compartment syndrome in other areas.
- Controversy exists in the amount of existing myofascial compartments of the foot.
- Multiple surgical approaches have been described for myofascial decompression.
- Controversy exists regarding acute versus delayed management of foot compartment syndrome.

J. G. Lugo-Pico
University of Miami Hospital, Department of Orthopedic Surgery, Miami, FL, USA

University of Miami/Jackson Memorial Hospital, Miami, FL, USA
e-mail: julian.lugopico@jhsmiami.org

A. Aiyer
University of Miami Hospital, Department of Orthopedic Surgery, Miami, FL, USA

J. Kaplan
University of Miami Hospital, Department of Orthopedic Surgery, Miami, FL, USA

Orthopedic Specialty Institute, Orange, CA, USA

A. R. Kadakia (✉)
University of Miami Hospital, Department of Orthopedic Surgery, Miami, FL, USA

Northwestern University, Northwestern Memorial Hospital, Chicago, IL, USA

© The Author(s) 2019
C. Mauffrey et al. (eds.), *Compartment Syndrome*,
https://doi.org/10.1007/978-3-030-22331-1_10

Table 10.1 Compartments and associated muscles of the foot

Compartment	Muscular structures	Location
Medial	Abductor hallucis, flexor hallucis brevis	Plantar medial to the first metatarsal
Superficial (superficial central)	Flexor digitorum longus Flexor digitorum brevis	
Lateral	Abductor digiti minimi Flexor digiti minimi brevis	Inferolateral surface of the fifth metatarsal
Adductor	Oblique head of the adductor hallucis	Plantar forefoot
Interossei (four compartments)	Each compartment includes the dorsal and plantar interosseous muscle of its location	Between each of the metatarsals
Calcaneal (deep central)	Quadratus plantae	

Foot Compartmental Anatomy

Early anatomic reports described four myofascial compartments of the foot: medial, lateral, central, and interosseous. Although surgical applications were previously based on these four compartments, recent research suggests the presence of nine myofascial compartments in the foot – medial, superficial, lateral, adductor, calcaneal [1, 2] – and four interosseous compartments [3]. Some authors describe a tenth compartment, the dorsal compartment, bounded by the skin which contains the extensor digitorum brevis and the extensor hallucis brevis [4, 5].

Table 10.1 shows compartments and associated muscles of the foot.

Etiology of Foot Compartment Syndrome

Foot compartment syndrome (FCS) is relatively uncommon, accounting for less than 5% of limb compartment syndrome cases [6]. It is caused by increased pressure secondary to hemorrhage or edema within an anatomic compartment. Ischemia results when this intra-compartmental pressure exceeds the capillary perfusion pressure [6]. It may be seen in the setting of high-energy injuries including crush mechanisms with and without osseous injury, Chopart and Lisfranc fractures dislocations, mid- and forefoot trauma, and calcaneal fractures [3, 7]. The most common cause of FCS is fracture of the calcaneus, accounting for 4.7–17% of cases [8–10]. This is likely in part related to the existing communication between the calcaneal compartment and the deep posterior compartment of the lower leg. Similarly, FCS can also be seen in tibia fracture and ankle fracture dislocations [11, 12]. Other causes of FCS include surgical procedures, occlusive dressings, frost bite, ischemia/reperfusion syndrome associated with vascular injuries, and exertional compartment syndrome [3, 5, 7, 13–15].

Clinical Evaluation

FCS is a clinical diagnosis, based on signs and symptoms of muscle ischemia. Classic clinical findings associated with compartment syndrome include pain out of proportion, paresthesia, pallor, pulselessness, and paralysis; however, these tend to be less reliable for evaluation of FCS than previously thought [6, 16]. Many types of injuries in the foot produce considerable pain; thus, pain out of proportion is not a reliable clinical finding in FCS. Pain with gentle, passive dorsiflexion of the toes has been described for diagnosing FCS; however, its utility remains questionable since this mainly tests the long flexor muscles which reside within the leg as opposed to within the foot compartments. Paresthesias can also be unreliable for diagnosing FCS because of the difficulty in determining whether the sensory deficits occurred secondary to nerve ischemia or to the initial injury. Palpable pulses (dorsalis pedis/posterior tibial) are usually present in FCS since the common sites for palpating foot pulses are extracompartmental; therefore, it is thought that vascular examinations are not sensitive enough to rule out the diagnosis of a compartment syndrome [3]. Several studies describe tense swelling as the most consistent physical examination finding in FCS [16, 17]. We have noted that tense swelling associated with severe pain not responsive to appropriate narcotic analgesia is a useful, though imperfect criteria in determining the presence of foot compartment syndrome.

While a through history and physical examination is the most important aspect to the diagnosis of FCS, it is not always clear if FCS is present. In this setting, the most objective means of diagnosing FCS is through compartment pressure monitoring [17–20]. This is particularly useful for diagnosing compartment syndrome in obtunded patients, patients with severe head or spinal cord injuries, or those who present with peripheral nerve injuries [3, 18]. Several techniques for compartment pressures measurement have described, but a commercial pressure monitor is likely the most reproducible, accurate, and easiest to use and is available in most hospitals [1, 2]. Due to the inconsistency regarding the anatomical compartments of the foot, there is no consensus regarding which or how many compartments' pressures should be measured. Currently, no evidence exists to provide a recommendation on how many compartment pressures should be measured in the diagnosis of FCS. The general consensus seems to be that the calcaneal compartment consistently demonstrates the highest pressures. Therefore, if pressure monitoring is utilized in the diagnosis of acute compartment syndrome of the foot, the calcaneal compartment should be checked [7]. Indications for treatment should be based on history/mechanism of injury, clinical findings, serial examinations over time, and a differential pressure reading between diastolic blood pressure and intra-compartmental pressure of less than 30 mm Hg [3].

Treatment Options

Initial management of suspected compartment syndrome includes the removal of all restrictive dressings, prevention of systemic hypotension, and serial examinations [18, 21]. Maligned osseous injuries of the forefoot/midfoot injuries should be reduced immediately. While reduction of calcaneal injuries may not be feasible, hindfoot dislocations should be reduced immediately if this is the suspected etiology of FCS. Additionally, the foot should be elevated to facilitate venous drainage, but not higher than the level of the heart to avoid compromising arterial blood flow [13, 18]. It has been described that a third of patients may develop FCS after more than 24 hours from the time of injury. Hence, in high-risk patients, serial examinations should be performed looking for signs of increased pain or until symptoms resolve [18, 21]. Once the diagnosis of foot compartment syndrome has been established, several authors recommend fasciotomies of the foot compartments [3, 11, 14, 18, 20, 22, 23]. Conversely, others do not consider the diagnosis of FCS to be an emergency and recommend against surgical management with the expectation of managing the sequelae of nonsurgical treatment [24].

Surgical Compartment Release

Multiple fasciotomy techniques have been described for the surgical management of FCS. The goal is to prevent ischemic contracture deformity of the foot and minimize development of neuropathic pain. The potential benefits of this procedure diminish the further out the decompression is completed from the time of diagnosis [6, 7]. Surgical techniques include the medial approach of Henry, combined medial and lateral incisions, two dorsal incisions, or a combination of these based on the underlying injury [3, 7, 18, 21, 25, 26]. A long plantar medial utilitarian incision has also been described [27, 28]. Currently, the three-incision approach is most commonly used, and it is based on the nine-compartment model of the foot. A medial incision is made 4 cm anterior to the posterior aspect of the heel and 3 cm superior to the plantar surface of the foot and is extended 6 cm distally. Through this medial approach, the media, superficial central, deep central, and lateral compartments are released. Two dorsal incisions are made to release the interosseous and adductor compartments. One incision just medial to the second metatarsal and one just lateral to the fourth metatarsal, this ensures an adequate skin bridge [6, 13, 28]. Overall, there are multiple fasciotomy techniques that exist for treating foot compartment syndrome, but no clear consensus on which technique provides the best patient outcome [3]. Additionally, the underlying nature of the injury as well as the potential for surgical intervention to treat the injury should be considered when planning incisions for compartment release, as specific placement of certain incisions is critical for definitive surgical treatment of these conditions.

Potential Complications and Sequelae

Surgical

Many authors recommend fasciotomy as treatment of choice for acute compartment syndrome of the foot; however, this is not without morbidity. After the fasciotomy has been performed, many recommend maintaining skin incisions open and performing secondary debridement, with or without the use of negative pressure wound dressing. This can be utilized until the swelling subsides enough for delayed primary closure or application of a split-thickness skin graft [3, 17, 18, 20, 22]. Even with this technique, the rate of superficial infection has been reported to be as high as 20%. Skin sloughing, necessitating split-thickness skin grafting, has also been described [20, 22]. In one study, near two-thirds of patients who underwent decompressive fasciotomy complained of pain, discomfort, and stiffness with ambulation at a 1-year follow-up, and 17% of patients developed postoperative paresthesias [17]. In addition, residual claw toe, injury to the medial plantar nerve, and severe scarring have also been reported [3]. Results have been variable with regard to quality of life after fasciotomy for FCS. In a prior retrospective study, only four of 26 patients who underwent foot fasciotomies were able to return to work [17]. However, most recent data reports that 78% of patients who underwent fasciotomies for FCS were able to return to work [29]. While these studies do provide outcome information after fasciotomies of the foot, the impact of the underlying bony injury on the overall patient outcome compared with the impact of the fasciotomy is unclear [3].

Nonsurgical

The goal of nonsurgical management is to achieve a functional, plantigrade, and painless foot. Potential sequelae include development of ischemic contractures, neuropathy, deformity, and chronic pain [11, 30, 31]. Ischemic contractures of the lesser toes can arise secondary to soft-tissue damage within the foot compartments and have been reported to occur within 13 months after the time of injury [11, 17, 28]. The type of toe deformity depends on the involved muscles, and the most commonly associated with contractures in the foot are hammertoe and claw toe deformity [3, 11, 18, 20, 28]. Hammertoes occur as a result of an imbalance between the extrinsic and intrinsic muscles of the foot. Due to FCS, the intrinsic toe flexors are weakened, thereby resulting in overpull of the flexor digitorum longus muscle. This leads to a flexion contracture of the proximal interphalangeal (PIP) joint with the distal interphalangeal joint in neutral or extension [28, 32]. Claw toe deformity also results from extrinsic muscle overpull against relatively weak intrinsic toe musculature (short flexors, interossei, and lumbrical muscles) [7]. This leads to extension of the metatarsophalangeal (MP) joint with flexion in the proximal and interphalangeal (PIP and DIP) joints. The key component in differentiating claw toes from hammer toes is hyperextension of the MP joint [32]. Neurologic deficit and chronic pain may result from injury to the posterior tibial nerve as it crosses near the calcaneal compartment [3, 11].

Controversies

Failure or delay to diagnose acute compartment syndrome may lead to irreparable soft-tissue damage and poor long-term function [3, 7, 22, 33]. Controversy exists regarding acute versus delayed management of FCS. Limited data exists regarding long-term outcomes of patients who develop an acute FCS. Many authors advocate toward emergent fasciotomy in attempts to improve blood flow by decreasing intra-compartmental pressures and prevent nerve-based pain; however, this belief is not universally shared due to the inherent risks of these procedures. Techniques for compartment release are inconsistent in the literature, likely arising from the debate regarding the number of foot compartments that exist and the compartments that are clinically relevant for decompression. To this date, there are no prospective, randomized trials comparing alternative approaches in the treatment of foot compartment syndrome. Further research on the outcomes of acute fasciotomy versus delayed management is needed. Patients must be counseled on the reported outcomes and potential complications of both surgical compartment release and nonsurgical management, thus allowing the patient to make an informed decision regarding treatment.

Take-Home Message
- Failure or delay to diagnose acute compartment syndrome may lead to irreparable soft-tissue damage and poor long-term function.
- Limited data exists regarding long-term outcomes of patients who develop an acute FCS.
- Near two-thirds of patients who underwent decompressive fasciotomy complained of pain, discomfort, and stiffness with ambulation at 1-year follow-up.
- Potential sequelae of nonsurgical management include development of ischemic contractures, neuropathy, deformity, and chronic pain.
- Patients must be counseled on the reported outcomes and potential complications of both surgical compartment release and nonsurgical management, thus allowing the patient to make an informed decision regarding treatment.
- If considering surgical FCS release, surgical approach should take into consideration definitive treatment of the underlying injury.

References

1. Matsen FA 3rd, Winquist RA, Krugmire RB Jr. Diagnosis and management of compartmental syndromes. J Bone Joint Surg Am. 1980;62(2):286–91.
2. Rorabeck CH, et al. Compartmental pressure measurements: an experimental investigation using the slit catheter. J Trauma. 1981;21(6):446–9.
3. Wells DB, Davidson AR, Murphey GA. Acute compartment syndrome of the foot: a review. Curr Orthop Pract. 2018;29(1):11–5.
4. Ling ZX, Kumar VP. The myofascial compartments of the foot: a cadaver study. J Bone Joint Surg Br. 2008;90(8):1114–8.
5. Andrew K, Sands SR, Manoli A 2nd. Foot compartment syndrome - a clinical review. Fuß & Sprunggelenk. 2015;13:11–21.

6. Middleton S, Clasper J. Compartment syndrome of the foot--implications for military surgeons. J R Army Med Corps. 2010;156(4):241–4.
7. Dodd A, Le I. Foot compartment syndrome: diagnosis and management. J Am Acad Orthop Surg. 2013;21(11):657–64.
8. Andermahr J, et al. Compartment syndrome of the foot. Clin Anat. 2001;14(3):184–9.
9. Perry MD, Manoli A 2nd. Reconstruction of the foot after leg or foot compartment syndrome. Crit Care Nurs Clin North Am. 2012;24(2):311–22.
10. Thakur NA, et al. Injury patterns causing isolated foot compartment syndrome. J Bone Joint Surg Am. 2012;94(11):1030–5.
11. Brey JM, Castro MD. Salvage of compartment syndrome of the leg and foot. Foot Ankle Clin. 2008;13(4):767–72.
12. Neilly D, et al. Acute compartment syndrome of the foot following open reduction and internal fixation of an ankle fracture. Injury. 2015;46(10):2064–8.
13. Fulkerson E, Razi A, Tejwani N. Review: acute compartment syndrome of the foot. Foot Ankle Int. 2003;24(2):180–7.
14. Murdock M, Murdoch MM. Compartment syndrome: a review of the literature. Clin Podiatr Med Surg. 2012;29(2):301–10, viii.
15. Younger A. Arthroscopic fracture reduction with fibular nail. In: Pfeffer MEG, Hintermann B, Sands A, Younger A, editors. Foot and ankle surgery. Philadelphia: Elsevier; 2018. p. 619–29.
16. Myerson M. Diagnosis and treatment of compartment syndrome of the foot. Orthopedics. 1990;13(7):711–7.
17. Fakhouri AJ, Manoli A 2nd. Acute foot compartment syndromes. J Orthop Trauma. 1992;6(2):223–8.
18. Myerson M. Acute compartment syndromes of the foot. Bull Hosp Jt Dis Orthop Inst. 1987;47(2):251–61.
19. Myerson MS. Experimental decompression of the fascial compartments of the foot--the basis for fasciotomy in acute compartment syndromes. Foot Ankle. 1988;8(6):308–14.
20. Myerson MS. Management of compartment syndromes of the foot. Clin Orthop Relat Res. 1991;271:239–48.
21. Frink M, et al. Compartment syndrome of the lower leg and foot. Clin Orthop Relat Res. 2010;468(4):940–50.
22. Brink F, et al. Mechanism of injury and treatment of trauma-associated acute compartment syndrome of the foot. Eur J Trauma Emerg Surg. 2014;40(5):529–33.
23. Giannoudis PV, et al. The impact of lower leg compartment syndrome on health related quality of life. Injury. 2002;33(2):117–21.
24. Wallin K, et al. Acute traumatic compartment syndrome in pediatric foot: a systematic review and case report. J Foot Ankle Surg. 2016;55(4):817–20.
25. Manoli A 2nd, Smith DG, Hansen ST Jr. Scarred muscle excision for the treatment of established ischemic contracture of the lower extremity. Clin Orthop Relat Res. 1993;292:309–14.
26. Myerson M. Split-thickness skin excision: its use for immediate wound care in crush injuries of the foot. Foot Ankle. 1989;10(2):54–60.
27. Loeffler RD Jr, Ballard A. Plantar fascial spaces of the foot and a proposed surgical approach. Foot Ankle. 1980;1(1):11–4.
28. Manoli A 2nd, Weber TG. Fasciotomy of the foot: an anatomical study with special reference to release of the calcaneal compartment. Foot Ankle. 1990;10(5):267–75.
29. Han F, et al. A prospective study of surgical outcomes and quality of life in severe foot trauma and associated compartment syndrome after fasciotomy. J Foot Ankle Surg. 2015;54(3):417–23.
30. Botte MJ, et al. Ischemic contracture of the foot and ankle: principles of management and prevention. Orthopedics. 1996;19(3):235–44.
31. Santi MD, Botte MJ. Volkmann's ischemic contracture of the foot and ankle: evaluation and treatment of established deformity. Foot Ankle Int. 1995;16(6):368–77.
32. Rammelt S, Zwipp H. Reconstructive surgery after compartment syndrome of the lower leg and foot. Eur J Trauma Emerg Surg. 2008;34(3):237.
33. Rosenthal R, et al. Sequelae of underdiagnosed foot compartment syndrome after calcaneal fractures. J Foot Ankle Surg. 2013;52(2):158–61.

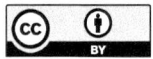

Chapter 11
Management of Missed Compartment Syndrome

Douglas W. Lundy and Jennifer L. Bruggers

Much has been written about acute compartment syndrome, and a recurring theme throughout the literature is that "the treating physician should never miss the diagnosis." Early diagnosis and treatment is a well-recognized factor that is integral to optimal outcomes after acute compartment syndrome. Unfortunately, many surgeons who are specialized in trauma care will see patients who present with a missed compartment syndrome. These patients may have had slowly evolving symptoms that persisted longer than the treating surgeon was aware in retrospect, or they may present with clear-cut missed compartment syndrome. In these situations, surgeons are faced with difficult treatment decisions and uncomfortable conversations with patients.

There are several reasons why a patient may appear with a delayed presentation of acute compartment syndrome. Unfortunately, many surgeons are often accused of medical negligence in these situations. Some patients may appear with a clinical picture that is unclear and have a slowly evolving compartment syndrome. Patients with perceived poor pain tolerance or a history of excessive opioid use may present with an acute compartment syndrome that can be difficult to diagnose. Poor communication with staff who fail to understand the alarming signs of compartment syndrome may also result in delayed diagnosis and subsequent treatment of acute compartment syndrome.

At times, compartment syndrome can be challenging to diagnose, and the signs and symptoms of this condition may be somewhat insensitive [1]. Ulmer [2] performed a meta-analysis of clinical studies of compartment syndrome patients and found that "the positive predictive value of the clinical findings was 11% to 15%, and the specificity and negative predictive value were each 97% to 98%." In response to these findings, he stated that "the clinical features of compartment syndrome are more useful by their absence in excluding the diagnosis than they are when present

D. W. Lundy (✉) · J. L. Bruggers
Resurgens Orthopedics, Atlanta, GA, USA
e-mail: lundydw@resurgens.com; bruggersjl@resurgens.com

© The Author(s) 2019
C. Mauffrey et al. (eds.), *Compartment Syndrome*,
https://doi.org/10.1007/978-3-030-22331-1_11

in confirming the diagnosis." Surgeons can often rest on this truth when they suspect that the patient is at risk for compartment syndrome but has not yet fully developed the condition. We can more reliably state that "it isn't there" than we can say "it absolutely is there".

Unfortunately, closed claim reports have documented cases of missed compartment syndrome where the treating surgeon seemed negligent in addressing the increasing signs and symptoms manifested by the patient. Although there are certainly situations when delayed recognition of the diagnosis may possibly be understandable, some cases just seem unexplainable. It is incumbent on the treating surgeon to anticipate acute compartment syndrome and be responsive when clear signs and symptoms present. O'Toole et al. [3] demonstrated that even highly trained orthopedic trauma surgeons in their Level I trauma center can have significantly different thresholds in diagnosing compartment syndrome. Recognizing that the diagnosis may be unclear and that delays in diagnosis may occur even in good systems, we should endeavor to make this unfortunate reality as rare as possible.

The hallmark symptom associated with acute compartment syndrome is "pain out of proportion." Patients who are sedated and intubated on ventilator support, head injured with a low GCS, or paralyzed from the spinal cord or other injury may be unable to communicate that they have severe pain, and the chance of missing the diagnosis of compartment syndrome increases significantly in these situations. Surgeons must communicate with staff to be very wary of acute compartment syndrome in "at-risk" patients and be vigilant for the signs of this condition. Clinical examination, to include increased pressure in the compartment upon palpation, pallor, and pulselessness, must be reported immediately to the surgeon. Recognizing that pulselessness and pallor may indicate that damage to the limb has exceeded the window for salvage, it is still extremely important for this finding to be communicated to the treating surgeons so that expedited treatment decisions can be considered. Certainly, no one wants to hear these findings as the first communication that a compartment syndrome is present, but the surgeon must consider the best options for the patient if this is the case.

Certain fracture patterns may forewarn the surgeon that the patient has an increased chance of developing a compartment syndrome, and the surgeon should have increased awareness of these factors in the patient that is difficult to assess. Auld et al. [4] found that AO/OTA type C forearm fractures were more likely to develop compartment syndrome than type A or B fractures. This study affirms the adage that extremities with fracture types associated with higher-energy injuries (such as comminuted patterns) also sustain increased energy in the soft tissue component, increasing the subsequent risk for acute compartment syndrome. Stark et al. [5] showed that medial tibial plateau fracture dislocations have a higher rate of compartment syndrome than the Schatzker VI tibial plateau fracture. Orthopedic surgeons should be extra vigilant when treating patients with injury patterns that are well-known to be associated with compartment syndrome.

An interesting injury pattern is the foot compartment syndrome associated with severe calcaneal fractures. Some surgeons believe that the treatment of foot compartment syndromes may in fact be worse than the sequelae of the syndrome.

Rosenthal et al. [6] found that the compartment syndrome patients in their series of calcaneal fractures had "toe clawing, permanent loss of function, persistent pain, muscle atrophy, contracture, painful warts, weakness, and sensory disturbances." They found that the patients with compartment syndrome reported functional outcomes that were significantly worse than those without compartment syndrome and that the Sanders III and IV fractures were the most likely to develop compartment syndrome. The pain associated with calcaneal fractures can be severe, and the surgeon should be aware that a compartment syndrome may exist in these situations. The surgeon should communicate the risks and benefits of fasciotomy with the patient and family so that they can make an informed decision regarding treatment.

Increased pressure to palpation in the compartment is a poor and inconsistent method to diagnose compartment syndrome, but this manifestation may be one of the very few clinical indicators left in the insensate or uncommunicative patient. Shuler and Dietz [7] examined the accuracy of orthopedic surgery resident's ability to estimate compartment pressures through palpation of the affected extremities. They found that the positive predictive value was 70%, and the negative predictive value was 63%. Although palpation of the limb and estimating pressure is not an ideal method for diagnosing compartment syndrome, there are situations when this sign may be the best that we have. Garner et al. [8] suggested that serial exams of the firmness of the compartments may be more sensitive in assessing for compartment syndrome, and they advocated that this may be a useful test in certain situations.

Advances in technology have not provided innovative and reliable methods to detect acute compartment syndrome. Shadgan [9] found that serologic studies are ineffective in the diagnosis of this condition. They found that creatinine kinase, myoglobin, and fatty acid-binding protein are elevated in injured patients as well as those in acute compartment syndrome, and these tests are insensitive in this regard. Wieck et al. [10] analyzed the ability of a polarographic probe to detect compartment syndrome by measuring differences in the partial pressure of oxygen in an animal model, but this has not been tested in human patients. This technology may have clinical application in the future.

Although most orthopedic trauma surgeons agree that the diagnosis of acute compartment syndrome should be based on the clinical presentation of the patient, the use of intracompartmental pressure measurements may be useful when assessing the insensate or obtunded patient. Collinge et al. [11] performed a survey of the Orthopedic Trauma Association and found that these assertions are widely accepted. Intracompartmental pressure may be considered as a part of the assessment of compartment syndrome, but these measurements should not stand alone as the sole decision point for treatment decisions. Intracompartmental pressure measurements are often unnecessary in the awake and alert patient, but they may provide valuable information in patients who cannot assess their pain and actively interact with the surgeon regarding decision making.

Indwelling pressure catheters providing constant measurement of compartment pressure have been shown to be ineffective in accurately diagnosing acute compartment syndrome. Harris et al. [12] found that 18% of their patients with indwelling catheters had a recorded Δp less than 30 mm Hg. None of these patients ever manifested a compartment syndrome, and none were treated with fasciotomy. The overall incidence of acute compartment syndrome in their study was 2.5%, and performing fasciotomy based only on reported increased pressure measurements would have been unindicated. Likewise, Prayson et al. [13] found in their study that 84% of patients had a Δp measurement less than 30 mm Hg and that 58% of patients had at least one measurement less than 20 mm Hg. None of the patients in their study developed a compartment syndrome. Ho et al. [14] measured the pressure in all four compartments of the leg at the beginning of surgery and immediately after reaming the tibia. They found that 23% of the patients had $\Delta P < 30$ mm Hg, yet none of them ever manifested clinical signs of compartment syndrome nor needed fasciotomy.

There are situations when a surgeon may accept a patient in transfer that has developed a compartment syndrome while in transit or still in the care of the referring physician. This can be extremely challenging since the surgeon often has no good information concerning when the compartment syndrome began and how far along the patient has been in the current condition. This is especially challenging in the uncommunicative or insensate patient. The surgeon has the dilemma of having to predict the future without the benefit of meaningful information about what has transpired. It is paramount in these situations for the surgeon to thoroughly communicate with the patient and family regarding the issues at hand and the risks of all decision pathways.

Consistent vigilance is required since recognition of a developing compartment syndrome is critical in performing fasciotomy within the acceptable window of time. In the era of resident work-hour restrictions and the proliferation of midlevel providers, it is understandable how communication errors can increase the likelihood of a delayed diagnosis of compartment syndrome. Garner et al. [8] describe an algorithm that could improve communication in treatment teams, thus decreasing the risk of missing a compartment syndrome. Their first step was to identify patients "at risk" and ensure that all members of the treatment team were aware of the concern for compartment syndrome. The second step was for the on-call resident or midlevel provider to perform compartment checks on the patient every 2–4 hours, and this person was tasked with communicating the findings to the team. The "compartment check" consisted of subjective pain assessment, reviewing the analgesic requirements since the last check and assessing the compartment fullness by palpation, passive stretch of the muscles, and a full neurologic and pulse examination.

Treatment

Orthopedic surgery residents are taught that compartment syndrome must be treated with fasciotomy. This is one of the few "always" statements in surgery, and violation of this rule is claimed to result in significant injury. The literature suggests however that this adage may not apply in cases of missed or delayed treatment of compartment syndrome. The available literature on missed compartment syndrome consists of retrospective case reports or series, and prospective randomized trials would be ethically inconceivable. Nonetheless, the available literature suggests that in certain situations, a missed compartment syndrome that has evolved past the acute injury phase may be treated nonoperatively in certain patients.

The surgeon must try to establish how long the ischemia has been present and how much damage is presumed to be present in the compartment. This determination is an extremely challenging process, and no one can consistently determine the clinical outcome in these cases. Nevertheless, an understanding of how long the ischemic injury has been occurring is very important in determining whether fasciotomy may prevent further damage or if that same procedure will begin the process toward amputation of the limb. All too often, a clear determination of ischemia time is impossible to determine, and the surgeon must make the best decision possible based off of limited and flawed data.

Glass et al. [15] performed a systematic review of the limited literature regarding missed lower extremity compartment syndrome. They identified nine studies that comprised 57 patients with missed compartment syndrome. They graded these studies as either "low" or "very low" quality. All but one patient in these reported series had emergent fasciotomy, and the subsequent amputation rate was alarming. They summarized that of the 63 limbs in the 56 patients that were managed surgically, 21 amputations were eventually required, and two patients died. The authors described the decision to perform emergent fasciotomy in cases of missed compartment syndrome as an act that "commits the surgeon to an amputation should the extent of muscle necrosis be unfavorable."

The same authors [15] performed a retrospective review of missed compartment syndrome at their facility commenting that this is a "rare and complex problem." They found ten cases of missed compartment syndrome resulting from delayed presentation, clinical error, or depressed consciousness that masked the presenting symptoms. They similarly had poor outcomes from surgical management of the first six cases, and anecdotally they managed the next four without surgery. All four of these cases were in individuals with compartment syndrome that affected one or two of the four compartments of the leg. All four of these patients seemed to fare better than the patients that had been treated with fasciotomy.

A reasonable question is "if there is significant ischemic damage in the compartment that leads to necrosis, how can nonoperative treatment be an option for these patients?" Glass et al. [15] stated that "ischemic damage depends on the magnitude of pressure, muscle mass, and metabolic requirements, the duration of delay does not correlate linearly with the pathological sequelae observed." Surgeons should carefully evaluate the patient and monitor for signs of sepsis or renal injury from evolving necrosis in the compartments. If there is concern that the load from ischemic damage is beyond the level that can lead to a satisfactory outcome without surgery, the surgeon must immediately perform fasciotomy and debridement understanding that this decision may lead to amputation.

The authors also stated that the decision to monitor missed compartment syndrome in lieu of fasciotomy should only be considered in the lower extremity. They advocate that missed compartment syndrome in the upper extremity should be treated with emergent surgery. Missed compartment syndrome in the upper extremity "represent a different clinical entity where preservation of fine motor function is of paramount importance."

Legal Issues

Unfortunately, missed compartment syndrome does occur, and it is a leading cause of medical liability claims filed against orthopedic surgeons [1]. Patient care must always be the center of our efforts and attention, but one cannot ignore the prevalent threat of medical liability litigation and the tremendous impact that it has on medical providers. While we must endeavor to always do what's best for patients, a consideration of the medicolegal risks is appropriate.

Bhattacharyya and Vrahas [16] examined 19 closed claims on 16 patients who sued their physician claiming negligence in the treatment of their acute compartment syndrome. The physician was victorious in 10 of the 19 claims, and all 3 of the claims that went to trial were found in favor of the physician. Not surprisingly, poor physician-patient communication and increasing time to fasciotomy more likely resulted in an indemnity payment. In their study, they found that fasciotomy within 8 hours of presentation of symptoms resulted in a successful defense.

It is vital for orthopedic surgeons to clearly document their findings and their thought processes when treating patients with suspected compartment syndrome. Defense attorneys prefer clear chart notes that elucidate that the surgeon was considering the possibility of acute compartment syndrome and their workup to rule in or rule out the diagnosis. While these chart notes can also be extremely helpful to communicate with other physicians and staff caring for the patient, they are extremely valuable in a medical liability defense years later.

Summary

An untreated compartment syndrome can be a devastating condition that can cause loss of limb or even life. Unfortunately, the diagnosis of compartment syndrome can be delayed or completely missed, and there are limited studies in the literature providing insight for treatment decisions. In certain cases, missed compartment syndrome may be monitored carefully by splinting the lower extremity in the functional position and observing the patient's metabolic and renal response to the injury. If there is concern for significant muscle necrosis, fasciotomy and debridement may be required, but this can often lead to amputation. Surgeons should endeavor to be hypervigilant to avoid missing a compartment syndrome in their patients.

References

1. Harvey EJ, Sanders DW, Shuler MS, Lawendy AR, Cole AL, Algahtani SM, Schmidt AH. What's new in acute compartment syndrome? J Orthop Trauma. 2012;26(12):699–702.
2. Ulmer T. The clinical diagnosis of compartment syndrome of the lower leg: are clinical findings predictive of the disorder? J Orthop Trauma. 2002;16(8):572–7.
3. O'Toole RV, Whitney A, Merchant N, Hui E, Higgins J, Kim TT, Sagebien C. Variation in the diagnosis of compartment syndrome by surgeons treating tibial shaft fractures. J Trauma. 2009;67(4):735–41.
4. Auld TS, Hwang JS, Stekas N, Gibson PD, Sirkin MS, Reilly MC, Adams MR. The correlation between the OTA/AO classification system and compartment syndrome in both bone forearm fractures. J Orthop Trauma. 2017;31(11):606–9.
5. Stark E, Stucken C, Trainer G, Tornetta P 3rd. Compartment syndrome in Schatzker type VI plateau fractures and medial condylar fracture-dislocations treated with temporary external fixation. J Orthop Trauma. 2009;23(7):502–6.
6. Rosenthal R, Tenenbaum S, Thein R, Steinberg EL, Luger E, Chechik O. Sequelae of underdiagnosed foot compartment syndrome after calcaneal fractures. J Foot Ankle Surg. 2013;52(2):158–61.
7. Shuler FD, Dietz MJ. Physicians' ability to manually detect isolated elevations in leg intra-compartmental pressure. J Bone Joint Surg. 2010;92-A:361–7.
8. Garner MR, Taylor SA, Gausden E, Lyden JP. Compartment syndrome: diagnosis, management and unique concerns in the twenty-first century. HSSJ. 2014;10:143–52.
9. Shadgan B, Menon M, O'Brien PJ, Reid WD. Diagnostic techniques in acute compartment syndrome of leg. J Orthop Trauma. 2008;22:581–7.
10. Weick JW, Kang H, Lee L, Kuether J, Liu X, Hansen EN, Kandemir U, Rollins MD, Mok JM. Direct measurement of tissue oxygenation as a method of diagnosis of acute compartment syndrome. J Orthop Trauma. 2016;30:585–91.
11. Collinge C, Attum B, Tornetta P 3rd, Obremskey W, Ahn J, Mirick G, Schmidt A, Spitker C, Coles C, Krause P. Acute compartment syndrome: An expert survey of Orthopaedic Trauma Association (OTA) members. J Orthop Trauma. 2018;32(5):e181–4.
12. Harris IA, Kadir A, Donald G. Continuous compartment pressure monitoring for tibia fractures: does it influence outcome? J Trauma. 2006;60:1330–5.
13. Prayson MJ, Chen JL, Hampers D, Vogt M, Fenwick J, Meredick R. Baseline compartment pressure measurements in isolated lower extremity fractures without clinical compartment syndrome. J Trauma. 2006;60:1037–40.
14. Ho KLK, Sing NYC, Wong KP, Huat AWT. Raised compartment pressures are frequently observed with tibial shaft fractures despite the absence of compartment syndrome: a prospective cohort study. J Orthop Surg (Hong Kong). 2017;25
15. Glass GG, Staruch RMT, Simmons J, Lawton G, Nanchahal J, Jain A, Hettiaratchy SP. Managing missed lower extremity compartment syndrome in the physiologically stable patient: a systematic review and lessons from a Level I trauma center. J Trauma Acute Care Surg. 2016;81(2):380–7.
16. Bhattacharyya T, Vrahas MS. The medical-legal aspects of compartment syndrome. J Bone Joint Surg Am. 2004;86-A(4):864–8.

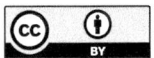

Chapter 12
Compartment Syndrome Due to Patient Positioning

Sascha Halvachizadeh, Kai Oliver Jensen, and Hans-Christoph Pape

Background

- Proper patient positioning is mandatory to provide optimal surgical access.
- Incorrect positioning is a risk factor for potentially severe long-term complications.
- Patients cannot communicate pain or other symptoms during surgery under general anesthesia.
- The lithotomy position can cause increased intracompartmental pressure (ICP) especially in the calf.

Epidemiology

One of the first and critical steps for any surgery is proper patient positioning. Its importance is often underestimated or performed by less experienced personnel. It is important to ensure adequate surgical exposure and optimal surgical access. Careful positioning also minimizes the risk of perioperative complications. Optimal perioperative positioning depends on the procedure and the surgeons' preferred approach. In the United States, 16% of surgically treated patients claim neural injuries while under anesthesia. In medical malpractice cases, injuries to the ulnar nerve (28%) or brachial plexus (20%) were most commonly claimed. Nearly half (45%) of these patients received a median payment of USD 35,000 for their claims [1]. Of these malpractice claims, 21.5% reported pressure ulcers due to inadequate surgical positioning [2]. The less physiologically the patient is positioned, the higher the risks for position-related complications.

S. Halvachizadeh (✉) · K. O. Jensen · H.-C. Pape
University Hospital Zurich, Trauma Department, Zurich, Zurich, Switzerland
e-mail: sascha.halvachizadeh@usz.ch

© The Author(s) 2019
C. Mauffrey et al. (eds.), *Compartment Syndrome*,
https://doi.org/10.1007/978-3-030-22331-1_12

An equally severe perioperative complication is compartment syndrome due to improper patient positioning. Its development is particularly dangerous because patients are unable to express pain and discomfort. Orthopedic and trauma surgeons are familiar with compartment syndrome treatment. However, other surgical specialties may only be confronted with compartment syndrome in the face of improper patient positioning of their own patients. Compartment syndrome develops most commonly in the calf. Prolonged positioning with intrusion of the forearm heightens the risk of development of a compartment syndrome. Further, one general risk factor that must always be considered is coagulopathy.

Positioning should maximize pressure distribution to avoid compression injuries to soft tissues or underlying neural structures. Every potential surgical position has advantages and pitfalls that medical personnel should be familiar with and consider when preparing for the procedure. This chapter serves to highlight specific risk factors in patient positioning for operative and nonoperative procedures in a variety of surgical subspecialties.

Compartment Syndrome

General Causes of Compartment Syndrome During Patient Positioning

In general, compartment syndrome is a result of decreased perfusion in a well-defined physiological space, associated with increased compartment pressure. Risk factors for the development of a compartment syndrome include the following:

- Prolonged direct pressure of the affected compartment. This scenario leads to edema, which increases compartmental pressure.
- Venous obstruction can elevate compartment pressures. Decreased venous drainage leads to extracellular fluid accumulation and edema.
- Insufficient perfusion. Diminished perfusion decreases tissue oxygen saturation leading to hypoxia, cellular edema, and ultimately cell death.
- Positioning of extremities alone can change intracompartmental pressures. For example, sustained dorsiflexion of the ankle physiologically increases intracompartmental pressure of the calf.
- Inappropriate fluid accumulation, for example, during misplaced/extravasal IV line.
- Increased bleeding due to coagulopathy.
- Duration of the procedure: After more than 5 hours of surgery, the risk of compartment syndrome rises significantly.

Surgeons must bear these considerations in mind during patient positioning for every individual procedure (Table 12.1).

Table 12.1 Summary of general risk factors in the development of a compartment syndrome during patient positioning or during surgical procedure

Prolonged surgery time (>5 hour)
Lithotomy position
Pressure on extremities
Vascular obstruction
Vascular procedures
Inappropriate fluid accumulation
Prolonged pressure
Hypoperfusion
Coagulopathy

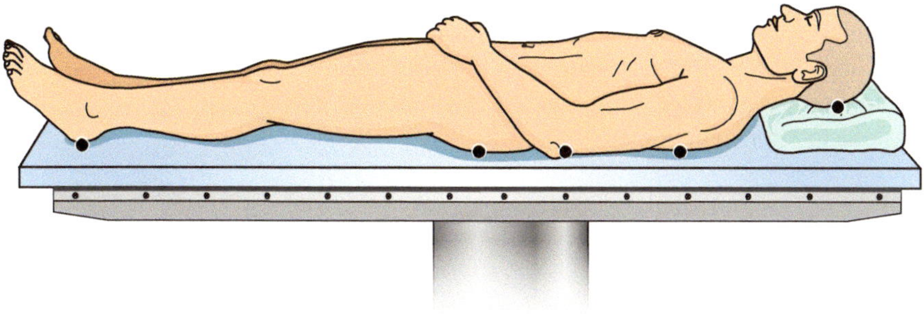

Fig. 12.1 Supine position with typical pressure points

Specific Surgical Positions Associated with Compartment Syndrome

Supine Position

Supine positioning is the most common surgical position and is the most physiologic position of an anesthetized patient (Fig. 12.1). Its advantages include ease of access to the abdomen, thorax, and extremities as well as the ease and speed of patient positioning. However, the supine position is subject to common complications including injury to superficial peripheral nerves and pressure ulcers. Injuries to the brachial plexus or venous obstruction in the neck due to lateral rotation of the head have also been reported. Acute compartment syndrome of the extremities rarely develops in the supine position. However, in prolonged surgeries or modified supine positioning, compartment syndrome has been reported. Positioning the limbs away from the body (such as 90° abduction of the upper extremity onto arm table) and subsequently fixating the positioned extremities pose the following risk factors:

- Pressure on the extremity due to fixation or a surgeon leaning against an extremity

- Extremities elevated above the level of the heart such as in angulated supine positioning
- Venous obstruction such as thoracic outlet syndrome

Lateral Decubitus Position

General complications of lateral decubitus positioning are similar to those found with the supine position (Fig. 12.2). The lateral decubitus position allows lateral approaches to the hip and the lower extremities. Moreover, it is used for certain spine procedures, some shoulder surgeries, and fibular bone grafting harvesting. In this position, the patient lies on the side with flexed hips and knees. The head should maintain a neutral position, and osseous prominences need sufficient padding. Prolonged discomfort raises the risks for subsequent complications. Similar to the lithotomy position, the lateral decubitus position is associated with the following risk factors for compartment syndrome:

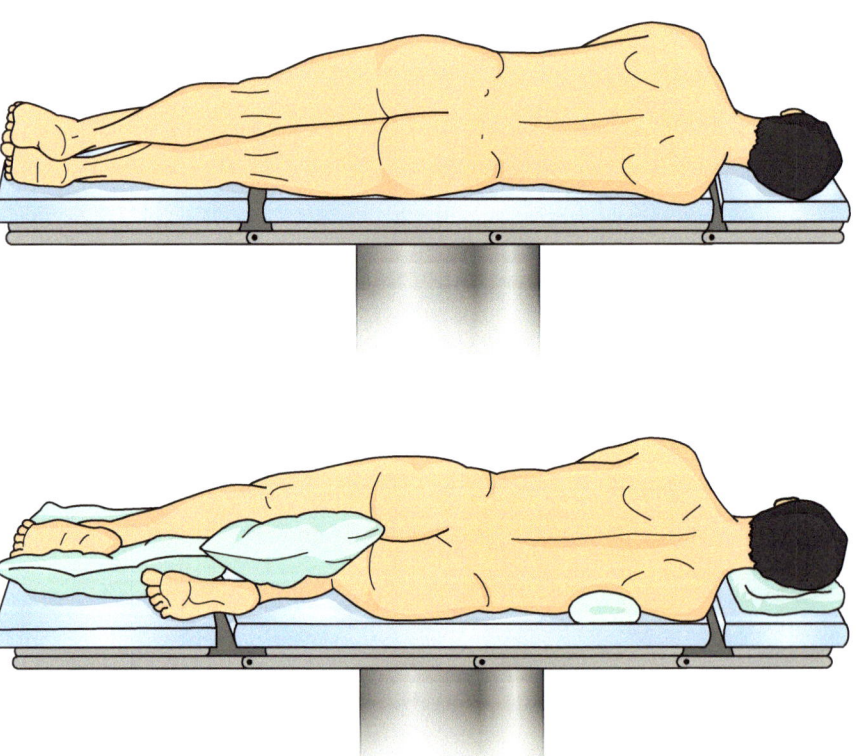

Fig. 12.2 Example of lateral decubitus position

- Pressure on the contralateral lower extremity
- Venous obstruction in the inguinal region due to hip flexion

This condition can lead to limb complications including ischemia, transient paresthesias, and rhabdomyolysis with the subsequent potential for renal failure. In one study, transient neurologic symptoms occurred after 5 hours and 45 minutes, with persistent neurologic deficits occurring after 8 hours. Another study that measured compartment pressures in healthy volunteers found that anterior tibial compartmental pressures in the bottom positioned contralateral leg could reach 240 mm Hg [3]. Compartment pressures of the anterior compartment of the bottom leg during compression by the upper leg showed elevated maximum average pressures of 57 mm Hg when padded on a soft surface and rises to an average 64 mm Hg on hard surfaces. The bottom upper extremity, compressed by the torso, showed maximum average compartment pressures of 100 mm Hg in the anterior flexor compartments. When the risk factors of pressure and vascular obstruction are combined, the risk of compartment syndrome rises significantly, especially in the bottom lower limb.

Prone Position

The prone position (Fig. 12.3) is one of the more complex surgical positions because it requires a high number of assistants to position the patient. Further, it requires increased anesthesiologic attention to ventilation and airway management, such as affirming proper endotracheal tube positioning by using mirrors. Prone spinal surgery may lead to bilateral superior iliac pressure ulcers. With respect to compartment syndrome, the following risk factors need to be considered when positioning the patient in prone position:

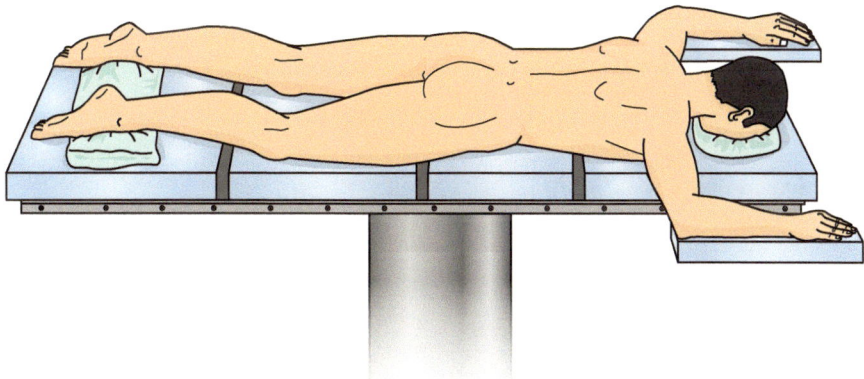

Fig. 12.3 Prone position: This position is more complex because it requires more personnel and higher anesthesiologic attention prior and during positioning

- Vascular obstruction in the inguinal region due to the patients' weight
- Pressure on the thighs
- Intra-orbital edema due to increased pressure in the fascial region

Fortunately, no wide-spread reports of compartment syndrome are available. One case [4], however, reported a compartment syndrome of the anterior compartment of the thigh after a procedure on the lumbosacral spine in prone position. Vascular obstruction in the inguinal region was postulated as the most likely cause of this complication. The combination of diminished inguinal blood flow and increased local pressure on the thigh in overweight patients raises the risk of developing compartment syndrome. Visual loss is also a known complication associated with prone positioning. Should a patient's head be positioned improperly on a soft headrest device, particularly if direct pressure on the eye is observed, the risk of orbital edema and subsequent compartment syndrome rises. While this complication is very rare, cases of ischemic orbital compartment syndrome have been reported in the literature [5].

Lithotomy Position

The lithotomy position is a supine surgical position that is most commonly associated with compartment syndrome. Surgeons use this position for optimal access to the pelvic and perineal organs (Fig. 12.4). The patient is placed supine while hips

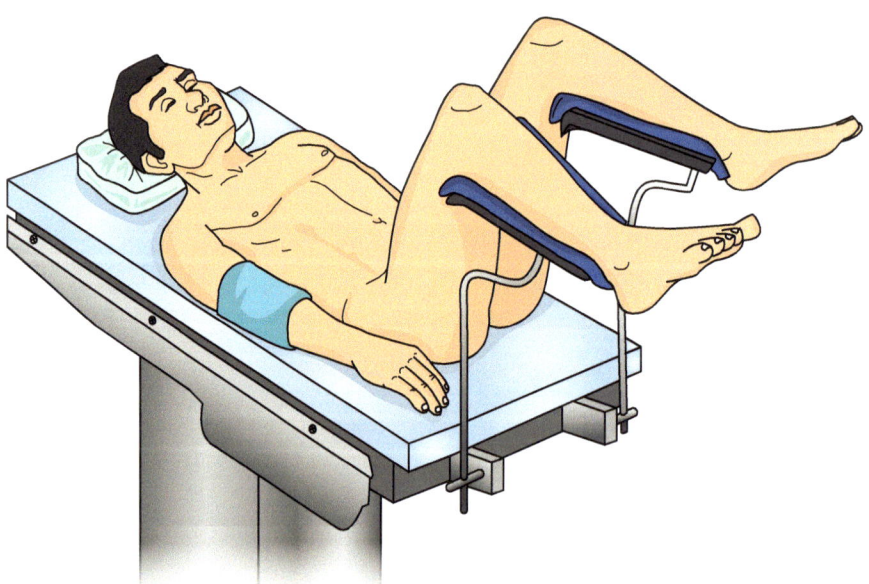

Fig. 12.4 Lithotomy position: During procedure, the surgeon gains good access to the perineal region. The elevated legs and the flexion in the hip are next to the pressure on the lower extremities considered as risk factors in the development of compart syndrome most commonly in the calf region

and knees are flexed as both legs are elevated. The legs are abducted, flexed, and elevated for adequate access to the lower abdomen and pelvic region. The most common complication associated with this position is neuropraxia of the common peroneal nerve (15.8%) [6] followed by compartment syndrome of the lower extremity.

The following characteristics of the lithotomy position are risk factors for the development of compartment syndrome:

- Pressure on the lower legs due to fixation of the legs on a support
- Legs elevated above the level of the heart
- Venous obstruction in the inguinal region due to hip flexion

The fixation of the legs produces increased external pressure, which subsequently causes intracompartmental edema, thereby raising intracompartmental pressure which may ultimately lead to compartment syndrome. Elevation of the legs above the level of the heart lowers local tissue perfusion, inducing hypoxia and producing edema or even tissue necrosis. In extreme cases, rhabdomyolysis and compartment syndrome result. Oftentimes, the lithotomy position requires hip flexion of at least 90°. Venous obstruction in the inguinal region may result, thereby lowering venous return, which allows interstitial fluid to accumulate, causing edema and increased compartment pressure.

Beach Chair Position

The beach chair position is characterized by Trendelenburg tilt of 10°–15°, 45°–60° of hip flexion, and 30° of knee flexion. Complications associated with this position include hypotensive bradycardic events, venous air embolism, hypoglossal nerve palsy, and neuropraxia of cutaneous nerves of the cervical plexus [7, 8]. Compartment syndrome risk factors include the following:

- Inguinal venous obstruction
- Pressure on the extremity due to fixation
- Elevation of the lower extremities due to Trendelenburg in modified beach chair positioning

In a case report of a laparoscopic robot-assisted cystoprostatectomy in modified beach chair position with Trendelenburg for 6 hours and total surgery time of 11 hours, Galyon et al. [9] reported compartment syndrome of limbs requiring fasciotomy. The etiology was postulated to be a combination of long duration of surgery, high BMI (33.9 Kg/m^2), obstruction of venous outflow in the lower extremity, hypoperfusion, and pressure due to fixation.

Gluteal Compartment Syndrome

While gluteal compartment syndrome has only rarely been reported in the literature, anatomic studies show that the gluteal musculature is compartmentalized. A systematic review of the literature found 28 cases of gluteal compartment syndrome

Table 12.2 Position-specific pathophysiologic response in the development of compartment syndrome

Lithotomy position	Elevation of the legs
	Pressure on legs due to fixation
	Vascular obstruction in the inguinal region
Lateral decubitus position	Pressure on the lower extremities on the nonoperated site
	Obstruction of vascular structures in the inguinal region
Supine position	Pressure on extremities
	Vascular obstruction in the neck
	Elevation of extremities in angulated supine positioning
Prone position	Vascular obstruction in the groin
	Pressure on the thigh
	Increased pressure in the facial region
Beach chair position	Inguinal vascular obstruction
	Pressure on extremities due to fixation
	Elevation of the extremity

reported in the literature with the most common cause being prolonged immobilization, accounting for 50% of cases [10]. Other major causes included trauma in 21% of cases and joint arthroplasty in the setting of epidural analgesia also in 21% of cases. Prolonged pressure on the gluteal area leads to hypoperfusion with subsequent tissue necrosis. Subsequent edema combined with venous obstruction raises intracompartmental pressure and increases the risk of developing gluteal compartment syndrome. Overall, risk factors include the following:

- Prolonged immobilization
- Epidural analgesia in the setting of joint arthroplasty
- Infection
- Trauma
- Vascular surgery
- Intramuscular drug abuse
- Altered level of consciousness (alcohol or drug overdose)

The position-specific risk factors are summarized in Table 12.2.

Intraoperative Diagnosis of Compartment Syndrome

Diagnosing compartment syndrome intraoperatively is challenging. The surgeon must be aware of major risk factors associated with the development of compartment syndrome including the following:

- Prolonged time of surgery (>5 hours)
- Lithotomy position
- Pressure on the extremities
- Inguinal vascular obstruction

If a compartment syndrome is suspected intraoperatively, the authors recommend measuring intracompartmental pressures with an ICP device while the patient is under general anesthesia. Normal physiologic supine intracompartmental pressure of an extremity at heart level is 5 mm Hg. Compartment syndrome is defined as an intracompartmental pressure 30 mm Hg greater than the diastolic blood pressure and serves as the threshold for surgical decompression of the compartment [11].

Therapeutic Recommendations

Therapy bases exclusively on decompression of all compartments of the affected extremity. The most effective and commonly used method is complete dermatofasciotomy (Fig. 12.5). We recommend protecting the fasciotomy with negative-pressure wound therapy (VAC), although a polyurethane synthetic skin substitute such as Epigard® may also be used. Secondary closure often follows about 5 days postoperatively depending on soft tissues.

Limitations and Pitfalls

The diagnosis of compartment syndrome is challenging, especially intraoperatively during general anesthesia, because patients are not able to express their symptoms. The lithotomy position is most commonly associated with the development of positional compartment syndrome. This position is mainly used for urologic and gynecologic procedures. Oftentimes, urologists and gynecologists are not routinely involved in treating compartment syndrome, as treatment is usually managed by general, orthopedic, or trauma surgeons. Physicians that are experienced in the

Fig. 12.5 Intraoperative documentation of an early compartment syndrome depicts immediately below the fasciotomy and swelling of the calf muscle as a sign of early compartment syndrome

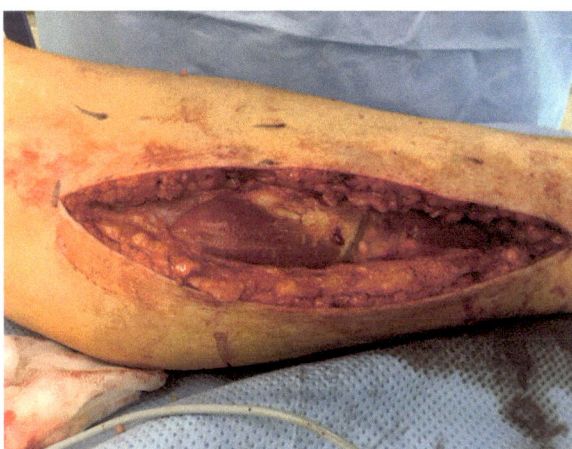

diagnosis and treatment of compartment syndrome should be promptly consulted if a compartment syndrome is suspected intra- or postoperatively.

While technical and digital advances in surgery provide huge potential for minimally invasive surgery with less surgical complications and morbidity, it is also associated with new complications. This case is especially true in robotic surgery (e.g., DaVinci) as the surgeon is not directly next to the patient. While focus on the procedure is high, the overview of the patient as a whole decreases, which potentially risks missing perioperative complications around the operating field.

Future Directions

Compartment syndrome due to surgical positioning is an uncommon complication, but can be associated with severe impacts on patient quality of life. The development of noninvasive devices for monitoring intracompartmental pressure intraoperatively and postoperatively represents a useful direction for future research and development.

References

1. Cheney FW, Domino KB, Caplan RA, Posner KL. Nerve injury associated with anesthesia A closed claims analysis. Anesthesiology. 1999;90(4):1062–9.
2. Schultz AA, Bien M, Dumond K, Brown K, Myers A. Etiology and incidence of pressure ulcers in surgical patients. AORN J. 1999;70(3):443–4.
3. Owen CA, Mubarak SJ, Hargens AR, Rutherford L, Garetto LP, Akeson WH. Intramuscular pressures with limb compression: clarification of the pathogenesis of the drug-induced muscle-compartment syndrome. N Engl J Med. 1979;300(21):1169–72.
4. Dahab R, Barrett C, Pillay R, De Matas M. Anterior thigh compartment syndrome after prone positioning for lumbosacral fixation. Eur Spine J. 2012;21(4):554–6.
5. Leibovitch I, Casson R, Laforest C, Selva D. Ischemic orbital compartment syndrome as a complication of spinal surgery in the prone position. Ophthalmology. 2006;113(1):105–8.
6. Angermeier K, Jordan G. Complications of the exaggerated lithotomy position: a review of 177 cases. J Urol. 1994;151(4):866–8.
7. McCulloch T, Liyanagama K, Petchell J. Relative hypotension in the beach-chair position: effects on middle cerebral artery blood velocity. Anaesth Intensive Care. 2010;38(3):486.
8. Valenza F, Vagginelli F, Tiby A, Francesconi S, Ronzoni G, Guglielmi M, et al. Effects of the beach chair position, positive end-expiratory pressure, and pneumoperitoneum on respiratory function in morbidly obese patients during anesthesia and paralysis. Anesthesiology. 2007;107(5):725–32.
9. Galyon SW, Richards KA, Pettus JA, Bodin SG. Three-limb compartment syndrome and rhabdomyolysis after robotic cystoprostatectomy. J Clin Anesth. 2011;23(1):75–8.
10. Henson JT, Roberts CS, Giannoudis PV. Gluteal compartment syndrome. Acta Orthop Belg. 2009;75(2):147.
11. McQueen M, Court-Brown C. Compartment monitoring in tibial fractures: the pressure threshold for decompression. J Bone Joint Surg. 1996;78(1):99–104.

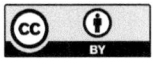

Chapter 13
Acute Compartment Syndrome in Children

David J. Hak

Compartment syndrome can occur due to a number of different etiologies, but most frequently occurs following high-energy trauma, which is less frequent in children than it is in adults. While the pathophysiology of compartment syndrome is the same as in adults, unique aspects of pediatric compartment syndrome include the challenges in examining and communicating with very young children. In addition, because the condition occurs uncommonly in children, providers caring for children may be unfamiliar with the signs of symptoms of patients developing compartment syndrome. While acute compartment syndrome in adults typically is observed to develop with the first 24 hours after injury, it has been suggested that the time between injury and development of peak compartment pressures may be longer in children [1]. Even longer times from inciting event or symptoms onset has been reported in children developing non-fracture-related compartment syndrome [2].

Epidemiology

Trauma is the most common etiology for the development of compartment syndrome in both children and adults. Additional non-traumatic causes of compartment syndrome include vascular injuries, surgical positioning, infections, and envenomation.

Compartment syndrome can affect children of any age. In children <10 years of age who develop compartment syndrome, the etiology is usually due to a vascular injury or infection, while in children >14 years of age, the etiology is usually due to trauma or surgical positioning [2–4]. Compartment syndrome occurs more commonly in males, especially adolescent males, and is associated with a higher rate of high-energy traumatic injuries in these patients who have a larger muscle mass [1–3, 5, 6].

D. J. Hak (✉)
Hughston Orthopedic Trauma Group, Central Florida Regional Hospital, Sanford, FL, USA

© The Author(s) 2019
C. Mauffrey et al. (eds.), *Compartment Syndrome*,
https://doi.org/10.1007/978-3-030-22331-1_13

Historically, compartment syndrome was most frequently seen in children with supracondylar humerus, forearm, and femoral shaft fractures [7]. Treatment of supracondylar humerus and femoral shaft fractures has changed over time, leading to a decrease in the associated incidence of compartment syndrome following these injuries. Supracondylar humerus fractures that historically were treated with closed reduction and casting in hyperflexion now undergo closed reduction and percutaneous pinning without the need to immobilize in hyperflexion. Femur fractures that historically were treated with 90-90 skeletal traction are now treated in a spica cast or with surgical fixation (flexible nailing or percutaneous plate fixation).

Currently, the most common condition causing development of compartment syndrome in children, as it is in adults, is trauma, resulting in tibial shaft fractures. Approximately 40% of pediatric compartment syndromes are due to tibial shaft fractures [4, 8].

Diagnosis

The diagnosis of acute traumatic compartment syndrome in children less than 5 years of age is especially challenging [1]. Very young children may not be able to accurately verbalize their symptoms, increasing the challenge in accurately diagnosing compartment syndrome. Young children may also have difficulty cooperating with the physical examination for compartment syndrome. While diagnosis is typically based on clinical examination findings in the setting of an injury placing the child at risk for compartment syndrome, measurement of compartment pressure may be required. This can be difficult or impossible in a young awake child and will often require some form of conscious sedation.

While the five Ps (*p*ain out of proportion or increasing in severity, *p*ain with *p*assive stretch, *p*alpable tenseness, *p*aresthesia, and *p*aralysis/motor weakness) remain a common criteria for diagnosing compartment syndrome in adults, a pneumonic of three As has been suggested for use in children. These findings include increasing *a*nxiety, increasing *a*gitation, and increasing *a*nalgesic requirements [9].

Tibia Fractures

Tibia fractures, especially high-energy injuries, represent the most common condition in which children develop compartment syndrome. In a review of 43 acute compartment syndromes associated with pediatric tibial fractures, 83% of cases were caused by motor vehicle accidents [1]. Development of compartment syndrome has been reported to occur in 4% of children sustaining an open tibial fracture [10]. A more recent review reported an 11.6% rate of compartment syndrome in 216 pediatric patients sustaining tibial fractures [3]. An increased use of compartment pressure measurement in this series may explain the higher rate of compartment syndrome diagnosis. Multivariate analysis in this study found that injuries due to motor vehicle accidents and children >14 years of age are at a higher risk for developing compartment syndrome. The rate of developing compartment syndrome was 48% in the subset of children >12 years of age with a tibia fracture due to a motor vehicle accident. In a large series examining the National Pediatric Trauma Registry, the incidence of compartment syndrome for open tibia fractures was 6.2% and for closed tibia fractures was 3.3% [5].

Tibial tubercle fractures represent a unique increased risk for the development of compartment syndrome in children. Associated injury to the anterior tibial recurrent artery can result in compartment syndrome of vascular compromise in as many as 10% of children sustaining tibial tubercle fractures [11].

A unique form of compartment syndrome centered in the region of the extensor retinaculum was reported in six children with distal tibial physeal fractures [12]. These patients presented with classic signs and symptoms of compartment syndrome including severe pain and ankle swelling, first web space hypoesthesia, extensor hallucis longus and extensor digitorum communis weakness, and pain with passive toe flexion. Compartment pressure measurements beneath the extensor retinaculum were > 40 mm Hg, while measurements in the anterior muscle compartment were < 20 mm Hg. These patients underwent release of the superior extensor retinaculum and stabilization of their fractures, resulting in rapid resolution of their symptoms.

Supracondylar Humerus Fractures

The reported incidence of compartment syndrome with contemporary treatment of supracondylar humerus fractures is only 0.1%–0.3% and most commonly involves the volar compartment of the forearm [13, 14]. While the volar forearm compartment is most commonly affected in cases of compartment syndrome following supracondylar humerus fracture, compartment syndrome involving the anterior arm, posterior arm, and mobile wad has also been reported [15, 16]. The diagnosis of compartment syndrome can be challenging in patients with supracondylar humerus fractures and median nerve palsy since the nerve injury may impair the child's pain sensation.

Increased risk of compartment syndrome occurs when supracondylar fractures are immobilized in greater than 90° of elbow flexion. Elbow flexion >90° was identified as a contributing factor in 8 of 9 cases of volar forearm compartment syndrome that occurred following closed reduction of a supracondylar humerus fracture [7].

Associated vascular compromise, in which swelling may be exacerbated during reperfusion, also increases the risk for development of compartment syndrome. In a series of supracondylar humerus fractures in which pulses were absent, compartment syndrome developed in 2 of 9 children without adequate hand perfusion, while no cases developed in 24 children with a pulseless but perfused hand [17].

Urgent treatment of displaced supracondylar humerus fractures had previously been recommended, but several studies have shown that an 8–12-hour delay in their treatment does not increase the risk of compartment syndrome [18–21]. Urgent treatment is still recommended for patients who present with a significant neurovascular deficit, and close monitoring is recommended in patients with severe swelling [22].

Forearm Fractures

Compartment syndrome has also been described in children sustaining both bone forearm fractures. In a large series examining the National Pediatric Trauma Registry, the incidence of compartment syndrome for open forearm fractures was 2.3% and for closed forearm fractures was 0.72% [5]. In smaller series, the incidence of compartment syndrome in children sustaining open forearm fractures has been reported to range from 7.7% to 11% [6, 23].

One study has suggested that extensive closed manipulation, as measured by length of operative time, increases the risk for development of postoperative compartment syndrome in children whose forearm fractures are treated by intramedullary nailing [24]. Investigators in this study reported the development of forearm compartment syndrome following intramedullary nailing occurred in 6% of open fractures and 10% of closed fractures. In comparison, they reported no compartment syndromes in 205 forearm fractures treated by closed reduction and casting. The use of a small incision has been advocated to minimize the amount of manipulation and facilitate reduction during intramedullary nailing of closed forearm fractures [6]. Using this technique in approximately half of their cases, they reported no compartment syndromes in 74 operatively treated closed forearm fractures.

Early surgical fixation may increase the risk of developing compartment syndrome. Two cases of compartment syndrome occurred in 30 children with forearm fractures treated with intramedullary nailing within 24 hours of injury, while none occurred in 73 patients treated more than 24 hours after injury [25].

Ipsilateral Humerus and Forearm Fractures

Children sustaining floating elbow injuries, ipsilateral distal humerus and forearm fractures, may have an increased risk for compartment syndrome. In one small series of nine patients, the incidence of compartment syndrome in this injury pattern was reported as 33% [26]. In another small series, two cases of compartment syndrome and four cases of impending compartment syndrome were reported in ten patients with floating elbow injuries in which the forearm fractures were treated by closed reduction and circumferential cast immobilization. In contrast, closed reduction and k-wire fixation of both the distal humerus and forearm fractures was safely performed in six cases without the development of compartment syndrome [27]. The increased swelling associated with this combined injury suggests that circumferential cast immobilization should be avoided.

Whether the floating elbow injury represents a significantly increased risk for compartment syndrome is questioned by a much larger series reported by Muchow et al. No cases of compartment syndrome were reported in this series of 150 cases of ipsilateral distal humerus and forearm fractures; however, they noted a higher rate of neurologic injury in the floating elbow injuries compared to that seen in isolated distal humerus fractures [28]. However, because there is an increased risk of nerve injury that can impair the diagnosis of compartment, increased vigilance for the possibility of a missed compartment syndrome is warranted in children sustaining a floating elbow injury.

Femur Fractures

The development of compartment syndrome has been described in young children treated with a particular 90-90 spica cast technique [29]. In most of these cases, a short leg cast was first applied and then traction was applied to the leg, and the authors speculated that this leads to impingement on the posterior compartment of the leg.

Neonatal Compartment Syndrome

A compartment syndrome-like condition involving the upper extremities that is thought to be caused by a combination of low neonatal blood pressure and birth trauma has been described and termed neonatal compartment syndrome [30]. This is a rare condition in which the diagnosis is often delayed [31]. A sentinel skin lesion of the forearm has been described as a clinical sign to identify this rare condition.

Non-traumatic Causes of Compartment Syndrome in Children

Although less common, it's important to understand that compartment syndrome can occur in the absence of fractures and remain vigilant in these scenarios of atypical presentation. In 12 cases of non-traumatic compartment syndrome, 10 patients were obtunded and treated in an intensive care unit [32]. The most common etiology was iatrogenic due to intravenous infiltration or failure to remove a phlebotomy tourniquet, and four cases resulted in an amputation.

Other non-traumatic causes of compartment syndrome include coagulopathy due to hepatic failure, renal failure, leukemia, and hemophilia [33–36]. Correction of the coagulopathy is necessary in conjunction with fasciotomy. Envenomation by snake-bites is another non-traumatic cause of compartment syndrome in children. The use of antivenin has been reported to eliminate the need for fasciotomy following rattle-snake bites in the majority of patients [37]. Exercise-related compartment syndrome can also occur, typically in adolescent males who are competitive athletes [2].

Treatment

External sources of compression should be removed in patients with an impending compartment and the limb maintained at the level of the heart (not elevated). Routine close clinical examination and/or compartment pressure measurement should be performed in these patients. Prompt diagnosis and fasciotomy is essential in avoid-ing tissue necrosis and functional deficits in patients with an established compart-ment syndrome. As described elsewhere in this textbook, the pressure threshold for fasciotomy is debatable. At least one study has found that normal compartment pressures are higher in children than in adults. In children, the mean compartment pressure of the lower leg ranged from13.3 mm Hg to 16.6 mm Hg, while in adults it ranged from 5.2 mm Hg to 9.7 mm Hg [38].

Summary

The diagnosis of compartment syndrome in children is primarily based on clinical examination and knowledge of injury pattern. Increasing need for pain medication fol-lowing a traumatic injury should alert the clinician to the possibility of compartment syndrome. Additional findings to consider in children include increasing anxiety and agitation. Compartment pressure measurement can be used in cases in which the diag-nosis is uncertain or in noncommunicative patients, but in children this typically requires sedation, and these values should be interpreted with caution since normal compartment pressures have been shown to be higher in children than in adults. Children with tibial fractures are at the highest risk for developing compartment syndrome, but several trau-matic and non-traumatic injuries can result in compartment syndrome.

References

1. Flynn JM, Bashyal RK, Yeger-McKeever M, Garner MR, Launay F, Sponseller PD. Acute trau-matic compartment syndrome of the leg in children: diagnosis and outcome. J Bone Joint Surg Am. 2011;93:937–41.
2. Livingston K, Glotzbecker M, Miller PE, Hresko MT, Hedequist D, Shore BJ. Pediatric non-fracture acute compartment syndrome: a review of 39 cases. J Pediatr Orthop. 2016;36:685–90.

3. Shore BJ, Glotzbecker MP, Zurakowski D, Gelbard E, Hedequist DJ, Matheney TH. Acute compartment syndrome in children and teenagers with tibial shaft fractures: incidence and multivariable risk factors. J Orthop Trauma. 2013;27:616–21.
4. Mashru RP, Herman MJ, Pizzutillo PD. Tibial shaft fractures in children and adolescents. J Am Acad Orthop Surg. 2005;13:345–52.
5. Grottkau BE, Epps HR, Di Scala C. Compartment syndrome in children and adolescents. J Pediatr Surg. 2005;40:678–82.
6. Blackman AJ, Wall LB, Keeler KA, et al. Acute compartment syndrome after intramedullary nailing of isolated radius and ulna fractures in children. J Pediatr Orthop. 2014;34:50–4.
7. Mubarak SJ, Carroll NC. Volkmann's contracture in children: aetiology and prevention. J Bone Joint Surg Br. 1979;61:285–93.
8. Bae DS, Kadiyala RK, Waters PM. Acute compartment syndrome in children: contemporary diagnosis, treatment, and outcome. J Pediatr Orthop. 2001;21:680–8.
9. Noonan KJ, McCarthy JJ. Compartment syndromes in the pediatric patient. J Pediatr Orthop. 2010;30:S96–S101.
10. Hope PG, Cole WG. Open fractures of the tibia in children. J Bone Joint Surg Br. 1992;74:546–53.
11. Pandya NK, Edmonds EW, Roocroft JH, et al. Tibial tubercle fractures: complications, classification, and the need for intra-articular assessment. J Pediatr Orthop. 2012;32:749–59.
12. Mubarak SJ. Extensor retinaculum syndrome of the ankle after injury to the distal tibial physis. J Bone Joint Surg Br. 2002;84:11–4.
13. Battaglia TC, Armstrong DG, Schwend RM. Factors affecting forearm compartment pressures in children with supracondylar fractures of the humerus. J Pediatr Orthop. 2002;22:431–9.
14. Ramachandran M, Skaggs DL, Crawford HA, et al. Delaying treatment of supracondylar fractures in children: has the pendulum swung too far? J Bone Joint Surg Br. 2008;90:1228–33.
15. Diesselhorst MM, Deck JW, Davey JP. Compartment syndrome of the upper arm after closed reduction and percutaneous pinning of a supracondylar humerus fracture. J Pediatr Orthop. 2014;34:e1–4.
16. Mai MC, Beck R, Gabriel K, et al. Posterior arm compartment syndrome after a combined supracondylar humeral and capitellar fractures in an adolescent: a case report. J Pediatr Orthop. 2011;31:e16–9.
17. Choi PD, Melikian R, Skaggs DL. Risk factors for vascular repair and compartment syndrome in the pulseless supracondylar humerus fracture in children. J Pediatr Orthop. 2010;30:50–6.
18. Gupta N, Kay RM, Leitch K, et al. Effect of surgical delay on perioperative complications and need for open reduction in supracondylar humerus fractures in children. J Pediatr Orthop. 2004;24:245–8.
19. Iyengar SR, Hoffinger SA, Townsend DR. Early versus delayed reduction and pinning of type III displaced supracondylar fractures of the humerus in children: a comparative study. J Orthop Trauma. 1999;13:51–5.
20. Leet AI, Frisancho J, Ebramzadeh E. Delayed treatment of type 3 supracondylar humerus fractures in children. J Pediatr Orthop. 2002;22:203–7.
21. Mehlman CT, Strub WM, Roy DR, et al. The effect of surgical timing on the perioperative complications of treatment of supracondylar humeral fractures in children. J Bone Joint Surg Am. 2001;83A:323–7.
22. Hosseinzadeh P, Hayes CB. Compartment syndrome in children. Orthop Clin N Am. 2016;47:579–87.
23. Haasbeek JF, Cole WG. Open fractures of the arm in children. J Bone Joint Surg Br. 1995;77:576–81.
24. Yuan PS, Pring ME, Gaynor TP, et al. Compartment syndrome following intramedullary fixation of pediatric forearm fractures. J Pediatr Orthop. 2004;24:370–5.
25. Flynn JM, Jones KJ, Garner MR, et al. Eleven years experience in the operative management of pediatric forearm fractures. J Pediatr Orthop. 2010;30:313–9.

26. Blakemore LC, Cooperman DR, Thompson GH, et al. Compartment syndrome in ipsilateral humerus and forearm fractures in children. Clin Orthop Relat Res. 2000;376:32–8.
27. Ring D, Waters PM, Hotchkiss RN, et al. Pediatric floating elbow. J Pediatr Orthop. 2001;21(4):456–9.
28. Muchow RD, Riccio AI, Garg S, et al. Neurological and vascular injury associated with supracondylar humerus fractures and ipsilateral forearm fractures in children. J Pediatr Orthop. 2015;35:121–5.
29. Mubarak SJ, Frick S, Sink E, Rathjen K, Noonan KJ. Volkmann contracture and compartment syndromes after femur fractures in children treated with 90/90 spica casts. J Pediatr Orthop. 2006;26:567–72.
30. Macer GA Jr. Forearm compartment syndrome in the newborn. J Hand Surg Am. 2006;31:1550.
31. Ragland R 3rd, Moukoko D, Ezaki M, et al. Forearm compartment syndrome in the newborn: report of 24 cases. J Hand Surg Am. 2005;30:997–1003.
32. Prasarn ML, Ouellette EA, Livingstone A, Giuffrida AY. Acute pediatric upper extremity compartment syndrome in the absence of fracture. J Pediatr Orthop. 2009;29:263–8.
33. Alioglu B, Avci Z, Baskin E, Ozcay F, Tuncay IC, Ozbek N. Successful use of recombinant factor VIIa (NovoSeven) in children with compartment syndrome: two case reports. J Pediatr Orthop. 2006;26:815–7.
34. Lee DK, Jeong WK, Lee DH, Lee SH. Multiple compartment syndrome in a pediatric patient with CML. J Pediatr Orthop. 2011;31:889–92.
35. Dumontier C, Sautet A, Man M, Bennani M, Apoil A. Entrapment and compartment syndromes of the upper limb in haemophilia. J Hand Surg Br. 1994;19:427–9.
36. Jones G, Thompson K, Johnson M. Acute compartment syndrome after minor trauma in a patient with undiagnosed mild haemophilia B. Lancet. 2013;382:1678.
37. Shaw BA, Hosalkar HS. Rattlesnake bites in children: antivenin treatment and surgical indications. J Bone Joint Surg Am. 2002;84:1624–9.
38. Staudt JM, Smeulders MJ, van der Horst CM. Normal compartment pressures of the lower leg in children. J Bone Joint Surg Br. 2008;90:215–9.

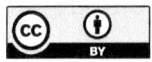

Chapter 14
Compartment Syndrome in Polytrauma Patients

Christopher Lee and Robert V. O'Toole

Background

Diagnosing compartment syndrome in the awake and oriented patient is difficult, and the diagnosis becomes even more problematic in the polytrauma patient. Many clinicians argue that the clinical signs and symptoms are the most important components in identification. Prompt diagnosis and treatment are just as critical in polytrauma patients for the prevention of long-term sequelae, including possible amputation. Unfortunately polytrauma patients who are often obtunded, intubated, and unable to cooperate with an examination, combined with painful high-energy injury to the limbs, create a very difficult environment for recognition of compartment syndrome. It is imperative to identify high-risk injuries and patients and to maintain a high level of clinical suspicion in those patients unable to participate in a clinical examination, and even then the possibility of a missed compartment syndrome is very real.

C. Lee (✉)
R Adams Cowley Shock Trauma Center, Department of Orthopedic Surgery, Baltimore, MA, USA

Virginia Commonwealth University, Department of Orthopedic Surgery, Trauma, Richmond, VA, USA

R. V. O'Toole
R Adams Cowley Shock Trauma Center, Department of Orthopedic Surgery, Baltimore, MA, USA
e-mail: ROtoole@som.umaryland.edu

© The Author(s) 2019
C. Mauffrey et al. (eds.), *Compartment Syndrome*,
https://doi.org/10.1007/978-3-030-22331-1_14

Recommendations

Prompt diagnosis of compartment syndrome remains the most integral factor to a successful outcome of compartment syndrome in polytrauma patients as it is in patients without polytrauma. Delay in diagnosis, and ultimately treatment of compartment syndrome, has been associated with permanent sensory and motor deficits, contractures, infection, and at times, amputation of the limb [1–3].

Physical Examination

Compartment syndrome has often been referred to as a clinical diagnosis, with various signs and symptoms postulated to be the most important or earliest presenting indicator. However, all of these clinical signs and symptoms require an alert and conscious patient, with a review of the literature suggesting a frequent delay in reaching the diagnosis of compartment syndrome as symptoms can be masked by other injuries in polytrauma patients [4–8].

Polytrauma patients have numerous risk factors for possible delay in diagnosis of compartment syndrome, including distracting injuries and altered consciousness. In the study by Frink et al., patients with multiple injuries and an Injury Severity Score > 16 had a mean time between admission and fasciotomy of 38 hours, in comparison with those patients with isolated injuries at 13 hours [9]. In those patients where altered mental status or pain evaluation is difficult to evaluate, the clinical signs of compartment syndrome become less helpful. Determining pain out of proportion that is expected for the injury, pain on passive stretch, paralysis and motor changes, and paresthesias requires a conscious and cooperative patient. Even in the setting of an alert patient with multiple injuries, determining the appropriate level of pain for a specific type of fracture is difficult. Pain can be influenced by psychosocial factors including anxiety, is of variable intensity, and is almost universal following any injury [10–12]. Furthermore, while increased analgesic requirements are important to assess, this is less reliable in the setting of multiple injuries and cannot be utilized in the presence of an unconscious patient. Paresthesia and paralysis are generally considered late clinical findings of compartment syndrome and cannot be evaluated in the unconscious patient.

The difficulty in performing a physical examination on an intubated patient is evident to all clinicians who have attempted this daunting task on a polytrauma patient. Take, for example, an attempt at physical inspection of swelling. Palpable and visible swelling are almost universally seen signs with acute compartment syndrome, but remain highly subjective even in an awake patient with an isolated injury. Assessment is routinely inadequate in polytrauma patients due to overlying splints and bandages and being inadequate to evaluate the deep compartments. Although sensitivity for this clinical finding is higher than other clinical signs and symptoms at 54%, the specificity (76%) and negative predictive value are far inferior (63%)

[13–15]. Furthermore, a physician's ability to manually detect isolated elevations in leg intracompartmental pressure has been identified as poor. In the study by Schuler et al., the frequency with which an anterior compartment fasciotomy was recommended was 19% when the pressure was 20 mm Hg, 35% when it was 40 mm Hg, 45% when it was 60 mm Hg, and 56% when it was 80 mm Hg. In the deep posterior compartment, it was 19% when the pressure was 20 mm Hg, 19% when the pressure was 40 mm Hg, 56% when it was 60 mm hg, and 64% when it was 80 mm Hg. When asked to qualify clinical interpretations of firmness as soft, compressible, or firm, participants descried the compartment as firm in only 45% of the cases in which the pressure was 80 mm Hg [16].

Risk Factor Assessment

As clinical signs and symptoms are of questionable utility in the setting of the intubated, unalert, or sedated patient, a high index of clinical suspicion is even more critical in the evaluation process of compartment syndrome in a polytrauma patient. This can begin with recognizing demographic factors and mechanisms of injury that place patients at increased risk for compartment syndrome. Perhaps the strongest predictor of compartment syndrome after a tibial diaphyseal fracture is youth, with the prevalence of compartment syndrome in adolescents and young adults 50 times greater than in those older than 60 years. Additionally, in the study by McQueen et al., the highest prevalence of compartment syndrome was between 12 and 19 years and 20 and 29 years [17]. This has previously been thought to be due to the relative size of the compartment and the muscle contained within it [17, 18]. In the studies by Court-Brown et al. and Shore et al., they identified adolescents sustaining high-energy tibia fractures as at-risk patients for compartment syndrome [19, 20].

Location of the injury can also help allocate patients into high-risk and low-risk groups. Compartment syndrome is most classically associated with tibia fractures, with rates ranging from 2.7% to 15% in the literature [18–26]. In particular, high-energy tibial plateau fractures have been associated with a greater risk of compartment syndrome, with associated fibular fracture increasing the risk [27–29]. The proposed reasons behind the relative increased risk of compartment syndrome in comparison with other aspects of the tibia include increased muscle proximally, the location of the nutrient vessel, and the robust venous supply around the knee. Additionally, in regard to tibia fractures, fracture length greater than 20% of the tibial length was found to be a risk factor for compartment syndrome in the study by Allmon et al. [27].

Furthermore, radiographic predictors of compartment syndrome can become very useful in polytrauma patients unable to participate in the clinical examination. In the study by Ziran et al., the displacement of the tibial anatomic axis from the femoral anatomic axis divided by the width of the femur at its widest point was a predictor of compartment syndrome in tibial plateau fractures. They found that a ratio of greater than 10% tripled the risk of developing compartment syndrome [30]. Additionally, ballistic fractures of the fibula and tibia have been associated with compartment syndrome. In particular, ballistic fractures of the proximal third of the tibia and fibula were at greatest risk for compartment syndrome among ballistic injuries [31].

Serum Markers

The use of other screening tools including specific biologic markers has also been explored in their utility in diagnosing or identifying an at-risk patient population for compartment syndrome. These objective measurements may be of particular use in the polytrauma patient, whose mental status may prevent clinical evalua-tion. In the prospective observational study by Kosir et al., patients who met high-risk criteria including pulmonary artery catheter-directed shock resuscitation, open or closed tibial shaft fracture, major vascular injury below the aortic bifurca-tion, abdominal compartment syndrome, or pelvic or lower extremity crush injury underwent a compartment syndrome screening protocol at admission and every 4 hours thereafter for the first 48 hours of admission. This screening included a comprehensive physical examination including lower leg circumference measure-ment, pain assessment, and vascular and neurologic examination, with any suspi-cious or unreliable physical examination findings mandating compartment pressure monitoring. No missed compartment syndrome was observed in the patients involved in this study, and the authors found during the first 24 hours of admission statistically greater base deficits (12.9 ± 5.9 mEq/L versus 7.5 ± 5.0 mEq/L), greater lactate levels (13.0 ± 5.2 mmol/L versus 5.4 ± 2.8 mmol/L), and greater PRBC requirements (28.4 units vs. 9.3 units) in those that developed compartment syndrome [32]. Other biological markers that have been associated with compartment syndrome include creatine kinase (CK) and lactate dehydrogenase. In patients treated with isolated limb perfusion, CK values exceeding 1000 IU/L after the first post isolated limb perfusion treatment day was correlated with compartment syndrome. LDH values peaked 2.9 days after CK values and was found to be less useful [33, 34]. In the study by Valdez et al., maximum CK greater than 4000 U/L, chloride levels greater than 104 mg/dL, and BUN less than 10 mg/dL were associated with the development of com-partment syndrome. When all variables were absent, no patients had compartment syndrome. When one, two, or three of these variables were present, the percentage of patients with compartments syndrome was 36%, 80%, and 100%, respectively [35]. However, this research was a retrospective study with limited patient num-bers, with future studies needed to validate these findings and correlate them with clinical examination. Furthermore, CK values may be of limited in utility in poly-trauma patients, as they can be elevated due to multiple injuries rather than the presence of compartment syndrome.

Intracompartmental Pressure Measurements

In addition to altered consciousness and other factors that interfere with history taking and assessment of physical signs, polytrauma patients, for various reasons, may have lowered diastolic pressures. This scenario could place these patients at increased risk for compartment syndrome as it can occur at relatively lower threshold pressures. Given the lack of clinical examination, the use of invasive intracompartmental pressure monitoring is appealing in this patient population. One of the first invasive measurement techniques used was a needle manometer, placed within the compartment and connected to a column filled with a mixture of saline and air, with the pressure calculated through the accompanying manometer [36–38]. The Stryker intracompartmental pressure monitor has been frequently used in North America, with current data suggesting optimal placement of the device within 5 cm of the level of the fracture but not at the level of the fracture [39, 40]. The anterior and deep posterior compartments of the lower leg have been most commonly advocated for measurement, as the anterior compartment is most frequently involved and the deep posterior compartment at increased risk for neglect [14, 22, 25, 39]. The threshold for decompression has undergone extensive deliberation, with the debate centered on using either the intracompartmental pressure alone or the differential pressure (ΔP). Studies have recognized that individual tolerance to absolute intracompartmental pressure varies widely and appears to be intrinsically associated with the systemic blood pressure or perfusion pressure [7, 15, 23, 37, 41–43]. As such, differential pressure has gained favor in determining thresholds for compartment syndrome. Clinical evidence and experimental data have suggested that a pressure difference of ≤30 mm Hg between intracompartmental pressures and diastolic pressure prior to anesthesia application should be a safe threshold for fasciotomy [25, 44–46].

However, the utilization of single intracompartmental pressure measurements may lead to overtreatment and unnecessary fasciotomies. In the study by Prayson et al., 84% of patients had differential pressures of 30 mm Hg with no clinical evidence of compartment syndrome [47]; however, this sample was small with disparate issues. In the study by Whitney et al., a consecutive cohort of 48 patients with tibia fractures and no clinical evidence of compartment syndrome at presentation found 35% of patients with differential pressures of 30 mm Hg [48], validating the general concern brought up by Prayson for a high false-positive rate with single pressure measurements. The Edinburgh protocol, which involved continuous pressure measurement and employing a ΔP of ≤30 mm Hg over a 2-hour period as the threshold for fasciotomy has been suggested as a means to reduce the time to fasciotomy while not significantly raising fasciotomy rates [25]. However, while clinical data seems to indicate that no compartment syndrome will be missed using a ΔP of ≤30 mm Hg as a threshold, this does not necessarily mean that this value signifies the presence of compartment syndrome.

Ultimately, current best practice includes high clinical suspicion and awareness. As polytrauma patients present unique challenges in the diagnosis of compartment syndrome, it is imperative to recognize at-risk patient factors and to understand the clinical tools available in conjunction with one another to diagnose compartment syndrome but also to understand the limitations of our current diagnostic tools in polytrauma patients. As has been shown, the use of isolated clinical exams, laboratory markers, and compartment pressure monitoring may all yield high false-positive results in polytrauma patients and perhaps lead to unnecessary fasciotomies. However, missed compartment syndrome is a potentially very serious situation. Hence, the diagnosis of compartment syndrome in polytrauma patients remains a difficult challenge.

Limitations and Pitfalls

With varying conscious states, limited participation in the clinical examination, and distracting injuries, polytrauma patients present a unique clinical challenge when diagnosing compartment syndrome. The drawback with using biologic markers and compartmental pressures with minimal clinical correlation is that these objective markers may be most useful in telling clinicians who does not need fasciotomy rather than who does. The inability to distinguish among traumatized limbs with true ischemic compartment syndrome in its early stages before tissue necrosis has occurred, those with impending compartment syndrome, and those with no compartment syndrome are in large part responsible for the lack of consensus on how to manage at-risk patients.

While some have advocated for continuous compartment pressure monitoring in the unalert, sedated, or intubated patient, continuous pressure monitoring remains controversial and infrequently used in North America. In the study by McQueen et al., the ability to close fasciotomy wounds at 48 hours was used as an indicator for unnecessary fasciotomy [49]. However, this remains a somewhat subjective and unvalidated way to determine if compartment syndrome was truly present. Most orthopedic trauma surgeons have experienced cases of complex fractures that are difficult to close but have no suspicion of compartment syndrome and evident compartment syndrome that can be closed immediately if they were released early. Thus, the utility of this definition to define true compartment syndrome remains open. It additionally appears that the use of continuous pressure monitoring may lead to increased rates of fasciotomy [50]. However, in a patient with distracting injuries and other factors that obscure the clinical picture, this may be one of the most reliable tools in preventing late diagnosis of compartment syndrome. Unfortunately, the most reliable indicator of compartment syndrome remains unknown, and currently surgeons must balance for themselves the possible risk of overtreatment with unnecessary fasciotomy against the potential clinical and medicolegal consequences of missed compartment syndrome.

An important limitation that applies to all human research in the field of compartment syndrome is the lack of a solid definition of compartment syndrome. The literature almost universally uses the performance of a fasciotomy as synonymous with compartment syndrome which creates great potential for research error given the known disagreement between surgeons on which patients have compartment syndrome [51]. This limitation is rarely discussed but is a major flaw affecting all of the human work in this domain.

Future Directions

Future directions for the diagnosis of compartment syndrome in polytrauma patients have focused on clinical labs or new sensors to diagnose and prevent compartment syndrome. Multiple new techniques to diagnose compartment syndrome are currently being developed and investigated in prospective trials [52].

One future avenue that has been explored was introduced by Odland et al. [53]. In this pilot study, a novel compartment monitoring system (CMS) catheter has two components: (1) one measures intramuscular pressure and (2) another removes excess tissue fluid. These catheters were inserted in the operating room after fixation of isolated tibial shaft fractures treated with intramedullary fixation in ten patients. This was done in conjunction with conventional Stryker catheters connected to the Stryker Intra-Compartmental Pressure Measuring Device. Intramuscular and blood pressure readings were recorded hourly for all catheters over a 24-hour observation period. They concluded that in comparison to conventional Stryker catheters, the CMS catheters were safe, had reasonable agreement in intramuscular pressure values with a high degree of correlation ($R^2 = 0.8$), and allowed for early and sustained reduction of intramuscular pressure with an average ultrafiltrate removal of 1.9 +/− 0.2 mL (1.2–2.7 mL). Additionally, the ultrafiltrate that was removed was analyzed for LDH and CK levels and was found to have a positive correlation between intramuscular pressure and enzyme level and a negative correlation between pulse pressure and enzyme level. Serum levels of CK and CK and LDH have been shown to be elevated but are not diagnostic for compartment syndrome [24, 25], and although low serum levels may mean no injury, low levels may also occur with severe injury and no perfusion. However, technology that will provide information about focal cellular metabolism or degree of cellular injury would be a significant advancement in the diagnosis and management of compartment syndrome.

Biomechanical markers have additionally been explored as a means of diagnosing compartment syndrome. Glucose, lactate, and pyruvate levels can detect muscle ischemia in situations of arterial occlusion, venous hypertension, and hypoperfusion [54, 55], and tissue glucose concentration was shown to detect ischemia within 15 minutes of vessel occlusion [56]. Glucose levels, as it relates to compartment syndrome, was studied in a canine model. In this study, interstitial glucose monitors were inserted into 12 canines, and acute compartment syndrome was created with mean compartment pressures of 74 mm Hg. Within 15 minutes of compartment syndrome, glucose concentration and oxygen tension were significantly decreased, and intramuscular glucose concentrations of less than 97 mg/dL was found to be

100% sensitive for the presence of compartment syndrome [57]. However, this has yet to be studied in traumatized human tissue, and the intramuscular component of the probe is too short to reach into a human tibial compartment. Nevertheless, this is one future direction that may allow for objective data to confirm the presence of compartment syndrome when clinical diagnosis is not possible.

A noninvasive avenue that does not require an alert and conscious patient has focused on measuring tissue oxygenation with use of near-infrared spectroscopy to determine the presence of compartment syndrome. Near-infrared spectroscopy utilizes differential light absorption properties to solve for the concentrations of oxygenated and deoxygenated hemoglobin through the use of the Beer–Lambert law [58–62]. Similar to conventional pulse oximetry, near-infrared spectroscopy utilizes light to solve for the percentage of oxygenated hemoglobin, although near-infrared spectroscopy can sample tissue as deep as 3 cm below the skin [58, 60, 63–66]. An initial animal study utilizing an infusion compartment syndrome model in pigs demonstrated an inverse relationship between near-infrared spectroscopy values and compartment syndrome [67]. In the study by Schuler et al. among 26 patients, six patients with unilateral tibial fractures in the absence of compartment syndrome had injured and uninjured limbs measured with near-infrared spectroscopy and compared these to uninjured control subjects. Results of this study showed a predictable increase in oxygenation of injured limbs by 15.4% points compared to matched uninjured contralateral limbs, demonstrating the body's increase in blood flow in response to injury [67]. In the subsequent study by Schuler et al., 14 patients enrolled after diagnosis of compartment syndrome both clinically and with intracompartmental pressure measurements were evaluated with near-infrared spectroscopy. Near-infrared spectroscopy values decreased by an average of 10.1%, 10.1%, 9.4%, and 16.3% in the anterior, lateral, deep posterior, and superficial posterior compartments, respectively. The authors postulated that these results suggest the clinician to be concerned about impaired blood flow to the injured limb should hyperemia in a patient with lower extremity trauma or fracture be absent [68]. Near-infrared spectroscopy could offer a means to evaluate the presence of absence of compartment syndrome in the intubated, unresponsive polytrauma patient. However, near-infrared spectroscopy values vary depending on skin pigmentation, and its applicability could be limited in patients with bilateral extremity injuries, and high-quality studies have recently been completed and await peer review publication to see if this technique is of clinical use [52].

Take-Home Message
The diagnosis of compartment syndrome remains a particularly challenging clinical entity in polytrauma patients. It has been well established that prompt diagnosis and surgical management of compartment syndrome provides the most optimal outcome for the patient. The diagnosis can become even more challenging in the polytrauma patient, where participation in the clinical examination can be limited due to altered consciousness, and

distracting injuries can complicate the clinical picture. Recognizing at-risk patients remains a critical first step. In particular, youth, especially between ages 12 and 29 years, appears to be a key factor for developing compartment syndrome, with tibia fractures being the most common precipitating injury. As regards injury, high-energy tibial plateau fractures with tibial anatomic axis deviation greater than 10% in comparison with the femoral anatomic axis, and ballistic injuries to the proximal tibia and fibula, remain high-risk fractures. Clinical markers including elevated lactate, large base deficits, elevated CK and LDH levels, and greater PRBC requirements should raise clinical suspicion in those patients unable to participate in the clinical examination. Finally, the use of serial compartment measurements in conjunction with the aforementioned findings can be helpful in the timely diagnosis of compartment syndrome. Future work is investigating measures of oxygen levels, glucose, lactate, and other local measures within the limb, but these are not yet in widespread clinical use and await validation. The authors currently advocate for the combined use of these clinical tools to diagnose compartment syndrome in the polytrauma patient, with the recognition that individual use of these tools can misdiagnose or overdiagnose compartment syndrome.

References

1. Muullett H, Al-Abed K, Prasad CV, et al. Outcomes Of compartment syndrome following intramedullary nailing of tibial diaphyseal fractures. Injury. 2001;32:411–3.
2. Prasarn ML, Ouellette EA, Livingstone A, et al. Acute pediatric upper extremity compartment syndrome in the absence of fracture. J Pediatr Orthop. 2009;29:263–8.
3. Rorabeck cH, Macnab L. Anterior tibial-compartment syndrome complicating fractures of the shaft of the tibia. J Bone Joint Surg Am. 1976;58:549–50.
4. Garfin SR, Mubarak SJ, Evans KL, et al. Quantification of intracompartmental pressure and volume under plaster casts. J Bone Joint Surg Am. 1981;63:449.
5. Lee BY, Brancato RF, Park IH, Shaw WW. Management of compartmental syndrome: diagnosis and surigcal considerations. Am J Surg. 1984;148:383.
6. Rorabeck CH. A practical approach to compartmental syndromes: part III. Management Instr Course Lect. 1983;32:102.
7. Rorabeck CH. The treatment of compartment syndromes of the leg. J Bone Joint Surg Br. 1984;66:93.
8. Sundararak GD, Mani K. Management of Volkmann's Ischemic contracture of the upper limb. J Hand Surg Br. 1985;10:401.
9. Frink M, Klaus AK, Kuther G, et al. Long term results of compartment syndrome of the lower limb in polytraumatised patients. Injury. 2007;38:607–13.
10. Matsen FA 3rd, Krugmire RB Jr. Compartmental syndromes. Surg Gynecol Obstet. 1978;147(6):943–9.
11. Eaton RG, Green WT. Volkmann's ischemia. A volar compartment syndrome of the forearm. Clin Orthop Relat Res. 1975;113:58–64.
12. Vranceanu AM, Barsky A, Ring D. Psychosocial aspects of disabling musculoskeletal pain. J Bone Joint Surg Am. 2009;91(8):2014–8.

13. Ulmer T. The clinical diagnosis of compartment syndrome of the lower leg: are clinical findings predictive of the disorder? J Orthop Trauma. 2002;16(8):572–7.
14. Matsen FA 3rd, Clawson DK. The deep posterior compartmental syndrome of the leg. J Bone Joint Surg Am. 1975;57(1):34–9.
15. Mubarak SJ, Owen CA, Hargens AR, Garetto LP, Akeson WH. Acute compartment syndromes: diagnosis and treatment with the aid of the wick catheter. J Bone Joint Surg Am. 1978;60(8):1091–5.
16. Schuler FD, Dietz MJ. Physicians' ability to manually detect isolated elevations in leg intracompartmental pressure. J Bone Joint Surg Am. 2010;92:361–7.
17. McQueen MM, Duckworth AD, Aitken SA, Sharma RA, Court-Brown CM. Predictors of compartment syndrome after tibial fracture. J Orthop Trauma. 2015;29:451–5.
18. McQueen MM, Gaston P, Court-Brown CM. Acute compartment syndrome. Who is at risk? J Bone Joint Surg Br. 2000;82:200–3.
19. Court-Brown CM, Byrnes T, McLaughlin G. Intramedullary nailing of tibial diaphyseal fractures in adolescents with open physes. Injury. 2003;34(1):781–5.
20. Shore BJ, Glotzbecker MP, Zurakowski D, Gelbard E, Hedequist DJ, Matheney TH. Acute compartment syndrome in children and teenagers with tibial shaft fractures: incidence and multivariable risk factors. J Orthop Trauma. 2013;27(11):616–21.
21. Mullett H, Al-Abed K, Prasad CV, O'Sullivan M. Outcomes of compartment syndrome following intramedullary nailing of tibial diaphyseal fractures. Injury. 2001;32(5):411–3.
22. Al-Dadah OQ, Darrah C, Cooper A, Donell ST, Patel AD. Continuous compartment pressure monitoring vs. clinical monitoring in tibial diaphyseal fractures. Injury. 2008;39(10):1204–9.
23. Blick SS, Brumback RJ, Poka A, Burgess AR, Ebraheim NA. Compartment syndrome in open tibial fractures. J Bone Joint Surg Am. 1986;68(9):1348–53.
24. Finkemeier CG, Schmidt AH, Kyle RF, Templeman DC, Varecka TF. A prospective, randomized study of intramedullary nails inserted with and without reaming for the treatment of open and closed fractures of the tibial shaft. J Orthop Trauma. 2000;14(3):187–93.
25. McQueen MM, Court-Brown CM. Compartment monitoring in tibial fractures. The pressure threshold for decompression. J Bone Joint Surg Br. 1996;78(1):99–104.
26. Williams J, Gibbons M, Trundle H, Murray D, Worlock P. Complications of nailing in closed tibial fractures. J Orthop Trauma. 1995;9(6):476–81.
27. Allmon C, Greenwell P, Paryavi E, Dubina A, O'Toole RV. Radiographic predictors of compartment syndrome occurring after tibial fracture. J Orthop Trauma. 2016;30:387–91.
28. Barei DP, Nore SE, Mills WJ, et al. Complications associated with internal fixation of high-energy bicondylar tibial plateau fractures utilizing a two-incision technique. J Orthop Trauma. 2004;18:649–57.
29. Egol KA, Tejwani NC, Capla EL, et al. Staged Management of High-Energy Proximal Tibia Fractures (OTA types 41): the results of a prospective, standardized protocol. J Orthop Trauma. 2005;19:448–55.
30. Ziran BH, Becher SJ. Radiographic predictors of compartment syndrome in tibial plateau fractures. J Orthop Trauma. 2013;27:612–5.
31. Meskey T, Hardcastle J, O'Toole RV. Are certain fractures at increased risk for compartment syndrome after civilian ballistic injury? J Trauma. 2011;71(5):1385–9.
32. Kosir R, Moore FA, Selby JH, et al. Acute lower extremity compartment syndrome (ALECS) screening protocol in critically ill trauma patients. J Trauma. 2007;63(2):28–75.
33. Shields RW, Root KE, Wilbourn AJ. Compartment syndromes and compression neuropathies in coma. Neurology. 1986;36:1370–4.
34. Vrouenraets BC, Kroon BB, Klaase JM, et al. Value of laboratory tests in monitoring acute regional toxicity after isolated limb perfusion. Ann Surg Oncol. 1997;4:88–94.
35. Valdez C, Schroeder E, Amdur R, Pascual J, Sarani B. Serum creatine kinase levels are associated with extremity compartment syndrome. J Trauma Acute Care Surg. 2013;74(2):441–7.
36. Matsen FA 3rd, Winquist RA, Krugmire RB Jr. Diagnosis and management of compartmental syndromes. J Bone Joint Surg Am. 1980;62(2):286–91.

37. Matsen FA 3rd, Mayo KA, Sheridan GW, Krugmire RB Jr. Monitoring of intramuscular pressure. Surgery. 1976;79(6):702–9.
38. Whitesides TE Jr, Haney TC, Harada H, Holmes HE, Morimoto K. A simple method for tissue pressure determination. Arch Surg. 1975;110(11):1311–3.
39. Heckman MM, Whitesides TE Jr, Grewe SR, Rooks MD. Compartment pressure in association with closed tibial fractures. The relationship between tissue pressure, compartment, and the distance from the site of the fracture. J Bone Joint Surg Am. 1994;76(9):1285–92.
40. Harris IA, Kadir A, Donald G. Continuous compartment pressure monitoring for tibia fractures: does it influence outcome? J Trauma. 2006;60(6):1330–5.
41. Halpern AA, Greene R, Nichols T, Burton DS. Compartment syndrome of the interosseous muscles: early recognition and treatment. Clin Orthop Relat Res. 1979;140:23-5.
42. Hargens AR, Akeson WH, Mubarak SJ, Owen CA, Evans KL, Garetto LP, Gonsalves MR, Schmidt DA. Fluid balance within the canine anterolateral compartment and its relationship to compartment syndromes. J Bone Joint Surg Am. 1978;60(4):499–505.
43. Allen MJ, Stirling AJ, Crawshaw CV, Barnes MR. Intracompartmental pressure monitoring of leg injuries. An aid to management. J Bone Joint Surg Br. 1985;67(1):53–7.
44. McQueen MM, Christie J, Court-Brown CM. Acute compartment syndrome in tibial diaphyseal fractures. J Bone Joint Surg Br. 1996;78(1):95–8.
45. White TO, Howell GE, Will EM, Court-Brown CM, McQueen MM. Elevated intramuscular compartment pressures do not influence outcomes after tibial fracture. J Trauma. 2003;55(6):1133–8.
46. Ozkayin N, Aktuglu K. Absolute compartment pressure versus differential pressure for the diagnosis of compartment syndrome in tibial fractures. Int Orthop. 2005;29(6):396–401.
47. Prayson MJ, Chen JL, Hampers D, Vogt M, Fenwick J, Meredick R. Baseline compartment pressure measurements in isolated lower extremity fractures without clinical compartment syndrome. J Trauma. 2006;60(5):1037–40.
48. Whitney A, O'Toole RV, Hui E, et al. Do One-Time intracompartmental pressure measurements have a high false-positive rate in diagnosing compartment syndrome? J Trauma. 2014;76(2):479–83.
49. McQueen MM, Duckworth AD, Aitken SA, Court-Brown CM. The estimated sensitivity and specificity of compartment pressure monitoring for acute compartment syndrome. J Bone Joint Surg Am. 2013;95(8):673–7.
50. Janzing M, Broos PL. Routine monitoring of compartment pressure in patients with tibial fractures: beware of overtreatment! Injury. 2001;32(5):415–21.
51. O'Toole RV, Whitney A, Merchant N, Kim T, Sagebien C. Variation in diagnosis of compartment syndrome by surgeons treating tibial shaft fractures. J Trauma. 2009;67(4):735–41.
52. Schmidt AH, Bosse MJ, Frey KP, et al. Predicting acute compartment syndrome (PACS): the role of continuous monitoring. J Orthop Trauma. 2017;31S(1):S40–7.
53. Odland RM, Schmidt AH. Compartment syndrome ultrafiltration catheters: report of a clinical pilot study of a novel method for managing patients at risk of compartment syndrome. J Orthop Trauma. 2011;25:358–65.
54. Setala L, Korvenoja EM, Harma MA, Alhava EM, Uusaro AV, Tenhunen JJ. Glucose, lactate, and pyruvate response in an experimental model of microvascular flap ischemia and reperfusion: a microdialysis study. Microsurgery. 2004;24:223–31.
55. Setala L, Joukainen S, Uusaro A, Alhava E, Harma M. Metabolic response in microvascular flaps during partial pedicle obstruction and hypovolemic shock. J Reconstr Microsurg. 2007;23:489–96.
56. Sitzman TJ, Hanson SE, King TW, Gutowski KA. Detection of flap venous and arterial occlusion using interstitial glucose monitoring in a rodent model. Plastic Reconstr Surg. 2010;126:71–9.
57. Doro CJ, Sitzman TJ, O'Toole RV. Can intramuscular glucose levels diagnose compartment syndrome? J Trauma Acute Care Surg. 2014;76(2):474–8.

58. Arimoto H, Egawa M, Yamada Y. Depth profile of diffuse reflectance near-infrared spectroscopy for measurement of water content in skin. Skin Res Technol. 2005;11:27–35.
59. Fadel PJ, Keller DM, Watanabe H, Raven PB, Thomas GD. Noninvasive assessment of sympathetic vasoconstriction in human and rodent skeletal muscle using near-infrared spectroscopy and Doppler ultrasound. J Appl Physiol. 2004;96L:1323–30.
60. Kim MB, Ward DS, Cartwright CR, Kolano J, Chlebowski S, Henson LC. Estimation of jugular venous O2 saturation from cerebral oximetry or arterial O2 saturation during isocapnic hypoxia. J Clin Monit Comput. 2000;16:191–9.
61. Mancini DM, Bolinger L, Li H, Kendrick K, Chance B, Wilson JR. Validation of near-infrared spectroscopy in humans. J Appl Physiol. 1994;77:2740–7.
62. Murkin JM, Adams SJ, Novick RJ, Quantz M, Bainbridge D, Iglesias I, Cleland A, Schaefer B, Irwin B, Fox S. Monitoring brain oxygen saturation during coronary bypass surgery: a randomized, prospective study. Anesth Analg. 2007;104:51–8.
63. Boushel R, Pott F, Madsen P, Radegran G, Nowak M, Quistorff B, Secher N. Muscle metabolism from near infrared spectroscopy during rhythmic handgrip in humans. Eur J Appl Physiol Occup Physiol. 1998;79:41–8.
64. Cui W, Kumar C, Chance B. Time-resolved spectroscopy and imaging of tissue. SPIE (The International Society for Optical Engineering). 1991;431:180–91.
65. Kaufman J, Almodovar MC, Zuk J, Friesen RH. Correlation of abdominal site near-infrared spectroscopy with gastric tonometry in infants following surgery for congenital heart disease. Pediatr Crit Care Med. 2008;9:62–8.
66. Schuler MS, Reisman WM, Whitesides TE Jr, Kinsey TL, Hammerberg EM, Davila MG, Moore TJ. Near-infrared spectroscopy in lower extremity trauma. J Bone Joint Surg Am. 2009;91:1360–8.
67. Garr JL, Gentilello LM, Cole PA, Mock CN, Matsen FA 3rd. Monitoring for compartmental syndrome using near-infrared spectroscopy: a noninvasive, continuous, transcutaneous monitoring technique. J Trauma. 1996;46:613–8.
68. Schuler MS, Reisman WM, Kinsey TL, Whitesides TE Jr, Hammerberg EM, Davila MG, Moore TJ. Correlation between muscle oxygenation and compartment pressures in acute compartment syndrome of the leg. J Bone Joint Surg. 2010;92:863–70.

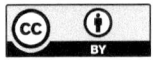

Chapter 15
Unusual Presentation of Compartment Syndrome

Ioannis V. Papachristos and Peter V. Giannoudis

Background of the Problem

- Compartment syndrome is a well-described clinical entity considered to be an orthopedic emergency affecting all ages.
- Prompt recognition permits expedited treatment which is paramount for a good outcome.
- The typical scenario for acute compartment syndrome (ACS) is lower limb fracture or crush injury. However, it has been shown that this is not always the case.
- There is a big diversity of systemic diseases, which can rarely cause compartment syndrome.
- Unusual anatomical locations, rare conditions, drug interactions, and their side effects as well as surgical procedures and rare fractures can also be associated with this syndrome.
- In this chapter, we will outline and analyze the various unusual forms where compartment syndrome can be encountered.

What Is Recommended

- Physicians need to be extremely vigilant when dealing with patients who could suffer from compartment syndrome.

I. V. Papachristos
Leeds Teaching Hospitals NHS Trust, Department of Trauma and Orthopedics, Leeds General Infirmary, Leeds, UK

P. V. Giannoudis (✉)
Academic Department of Trauma and Orthopedics, School of Medicine, University of Leeds, NIHR Leeds Biomedical Research Center, Chapel Allerton Hospital, Leeds Teaching Hospitals NHS Trust, Leeds, UK
e-mail: peter.giannoudis@nhs.net

© The Author(s) 2019
C. Mauffrey et al. (eds.), *Compartment Syndrome*,
https://doi.org/10.1007/978-3-030-22331-1_15

- Good knowledge of its pathophysiology will help the surgeon guide his thought toward the specific diagnosis even in unusual presentations escaping from this difficult clinical setting.
- Awareness of unusual presentations, causes, or scenarios which can hide compartment syndrome should be known. The scope of this chapter is to increase the awareness of these situations.

Limitations and Pitfalls

This study is a detailed outline and analysis of a variety of rare presentations of compartment syndrome. It is impossible to include all the possible eventualities where a compartment syndrome can occur. We performed an extensive review of the available literature, but we acknowledge that there may be limited cases or conditions we may not have mentioned.

Future Directions

Further research is needed regarding diagnostic measures of compartment syndrome. More publications will give us further insight to this diverse problem.

Introduction

Compartment syndrome is characterized by an increase in pressure in a contained fibro-osseous compartment, such as the forearm or leg, resulting sequentially in decreased lymphatic and venous drainage, loss of arterial inflow, and subsequently diminishing of perfusion pressure. This leads to neuromuscular hypoxia and death of the contained structures. Established compartment syndrome if left untreated leads to contractures, sensory deficits, paralysis, permanent disability, amputation, and even death. In order to minimize morbidity and optimize treatment of a patient at risk for compartment syndrome, clinicians need a clear understanding of the pathophysiology, means (and problems) of diagnosis, and treatment of compartment syndrome. The typical scenario of compartment syndrome involves a young male with lower limb fracture or severe injury and presenting with tight leg compartments and pain out of proportion which cannot be relieved by painkillers. However, there is a great diversity of unusual conditions, common systemic diseases, medications, procedures, and atypical circumstances, which can be complicated by compartment syndrome.

Unusual Conditions

Exertional compartment syndrome is caused when strenuous exercise leads to swelling of the overexerted muscle in a closed compartment, resulting in increased tissue pressure. Wilson was the first to describe this uncommon type of compartment syndrome in 1912, and later Vogt in 1945 termed it as "march gangrene" [1]. Compartment syndrome after exercise can be divided in acute, acute-on-chronic or chronic, depending on the emergency or not of its presentation [2]. It was initially thought to affect only athletes, but Edmundsson et al. in 2007 reported that 36 out of 73 nonathletic referred patients suffering from exercise-induced pain were suffering from chronic compartment syndrome [3]. Exertional compartment syndrome has been frequently reported in people who follow a sedentary way of life and enthusiastically participate in intense sports activities.

Livingston et al. published this year a descriptive case series of seven young athletes suffering from acute exertional compartment syndrome (AECS) of lower leg [4]. In their retrospective study, they compared young athletes who suffered ACS after exertion with similar patients after a fracture. Diagnosis was set on average after 97 hours from symptom onset, whereas for fracture group this was 19 hours and only one patient required release of four compartments. Five out of seven patients had full recovery, whereas the other two needed a form of ankle orthosis. They postulated that half of those with longer than 24 hours of symptoms suffered from substantial muscle necrosis and functional deficit at final follow-up. In contrast, when the diagnosis of AECS was made in less than 24 hours of symptoms, there was no evidence of long-term sequelae. They also highlighted that patients with AECS were able to weightbear which complicates diagnosis as clinicians are trained to believe that pain from ACS precludes weightbearing. On their series, 86% exhibited neurologic deficit compared to 20% of fracture ACS, showing that neurologic damage is already present upon diagnosis. In AECS, anterior and lateral tibial compartments are mostly affected than the posterior compartments, and this phenomenon can be attributed to the fact that anterior tibialis and peroneus longus have higher percentage of fast-twitch fibers, making them prone to ischemia, whereas posterior compartment muscles have higher percentage of slow-twitch fibers, making them resistant to ischemia and suitable for endurance [5]. However, in Livingston's series, despite the high average intracompartmental pressures measured (91 mm Hg), there was no correlation between pressure and muscle damage, but a strong correlation of a time to diagnose more than 24 hours and myonecrosis is evident. This year, McKinney et al. reported a case of AECS affecting the anterior tibial compartment presenting with foot drop which was successfully treated with anterior lateral fasciotomies and rhabdomyolysis-supportive treatment, giving him full recovery apart from inability to extend of his hallux due to EHL necrosis [6]. Nicholson et al. reported AECS of the peroneal compartment on a 24-year-old healthy female after prolonged horse riding [7]. This was the first case related to a non-ground sporting activity. The patient presented with sensory deficit on the first web space and dorsum of the foot, peroneal inability, and pain on anterolateral compartment, and this compartment was found to be necrotic during four-compartment fasciotomy. Common peroneal nerve, anterior tibialis muscle, and two other compartments were found healthy. Eventually, she made an excellent recovery, and authors postulated that this happened to her right leg due to the high boots and the leg position (knee flexed and dorsiflexed/inverted ankle) and not in the contralateral owing to a possible anatomical difference. Medial gastrocnemius tear was reported as a cause of AECS in a 55-year-old man who was running to catch a bus [8]. Four-compartment release showed the medial gastrocnemius tear 15 mm distal to the knee along with tear in peroneal artery and the resultant hematoma. Moreover, AECS can affect the upper limbs. In 2014, Bunting et al. reported bilateral supraspinatus AECS on a healthy 23-year-old male after strenuous weight lifting for an extended period [9]. Ultrasound-guided intracompartmental pressure measurements depicted pressures of 24 and 25 mmHg on the left and right trapezius, respectively, as well as 56 and 85 mmHg for left and right supraspinatus, respectively. With normal pressures considered to be from 3 to 20 mmHg, the diagnosis of bilateral supraspinatus AECS was set, and fasciotomies offered complete relief and excellent recovery.

Chronic exertional compartment syndrome (CECS) represents the result of overuse injuries affecting the extremities. The leg is the most frequent anatomical site particularly in running athletes [10]. CECS represents the second most common cause of exertional leg pain after medial tibial stress syndrome with an incidence ranging from 27% to 33% [11]. It appears equally in men and women at an average age of 20 [12]. The most commonly affected compartments are the anterior and lateral compartments (or a combination thereof) with an incidence of up to 95% of all CECS [13]. Typically, patients present with symptoms after increased intensity and duration of workouts that abate with cessation of activity. Over time, the pain that is experienced during exercise may increase, and patients may experience greater limitations during the provoking activities. Since symptoms are alleviated at rest, the ailment can frequently go undiagnosed for a period of time, increasing the severity of the condition. CECS is a clinical diagnosis; however objective measurements of intracompartmental pressures aid in confirming the diagnosis [14]. During exertion, compartment pressures increase three or four times from the baseline and return to basal levels within a few minutes in normal patients, whereas in patients with CECS, pressures increase more strikingly and take longer to return to their baseline (over 10 minutes) [15]. Pedowitz et al. in 1990 published modified criteria for the diagnosis of CECS based on intracompartmental pressures as up to then there was no consensus in the literature [16]. The criteria were based upon the intramuscular pressures recorded with the slit catheter before and after exercise in 210 muscle compartments without CECS. In the presence of appropriate clinical findings, they stated one or more of the following intramuscular pressure criteria to be diagnostic of chronic compartment syndrome of the leg: (1) a pre-exercise pressure greater than or equal to 15 mm Hg, (2) a 1-minute post-exercise pressure of greater than or equal to 30 mm Hg, or (3) a 5-minute post-exercise pressure greater than or equal to 20 mm Hg. Application of these criteria should result in a less than 5%

incidence of false-positive diagnoses. The only significant clinical difference between the group of patients suffering from CECS and non-CECS ones was muscle hernia at an incidence of 45.9% versus 12.9%, respectively. However, in 2012 Roberts et al. questioned the validity of these criteria [17]. They reviewed 38 studies from 1966 to 2010 and concluded that if clinicians carry out IMP testing, they should use a protocol with standardized catheter depth, exercise type, intensity and duration, footwear, and equipment. They argued that with the exception of relaxation pressure, the criteria set by Pedowitz for diagnosing CECS, considered to be the gold standard, overlapped the range found in normal healthy subjects. Therefore, they concluded that maximum reported upper confidence limits for pre, during, relaxation, and post 1- and 5-minute IMPs are 32 mmHg, 98 mmHg, 59 mmHg, 69 mmHg, and 48 mmHg, respectively. Pressures above these maximum values could certainly be considered abnormal under any circumstance. Although guaranteeing high specificity, the use of these values as cutoffs would likely have severe consequences on sensitivity. Therefore, they stated that mean upper confidence limits for the five time points are 14 mmHg (pre-exercise), 54 mmHg (during), 18 mmHg (relaxation), 36 mmHg (post 1 minute), and 23 mmHg (post 5 minutes). Values more than these must always be combined with clinical evaluation to safely reach a diagnosis. Nonoperative treatment of CECS includes rest, removal from inciting activity, stretching, anti-inflammatories, correction of training errors, and orthotics. However, this treatment is rarely followed due to the intensity of symptoms and also because patients cannot afford to abstain from their activities. Release of the anterior and lateral compartments has predicable success rates of roughly 80%, while deep posterior releases may yield success rates of 50% [18]. Irion et al. on their case series of 13 elite-level young athletes reported an 84.6% rate of return to their prior-activity level after an average of 10.6 weeks following surgical fasciectomy for CECS [10]. Involvement of four compartments resulted in longer return to full sporting activities after release. In a review of 100 fasciotomies for CECS, Detmer reported a recurrence rate of 3.4% [19]. CECS affecting the forearm usually involves the flexor compartment because of the higher exertion applied on these muscles during sporting activity and often occurs in rowers, climbers, and gymnasts. Open fasciotomies are considered the treatment of choice for forearm CECS, and these are the recommended ones. Nonetheless, endoscopic technique with single or multiple portals has also been described [20].

Neonatal form of compartment syndrome is rare and usually affects the forearm, wrist, and hand. The initial presentation is a superficial sentinel skin lesion or "sucking blister" at birth [21]. Several compression factors and neonatal conditions can induce neonatal compartment syndrome. Local mechanical causes include umbilical cord loops, fetal posture and oligoamnios, twin pregnancy, maternal uterine malformation, and amniotic band constriction [22]. This mechanical compression can be accentuated by maternal and neonatal conditions such as respiratory distress, vascular insufficiency, clotting disorders, and maternal diabetes [23]. It should be distinguished from gangrene of the newborn (usually involves lower limbs) [24], from necrotizing fasciitis (fulminating course of sepsis and skin lesions), and from aplasia cutis congenital (congenital absence of skin; ulcers involving symmetrical scalp, trunk, and extremities; and heal spontaneously) [25]. The time from birth to surgery is the main prognostic factor. Misdiagnosis may lead to muscular and neuronal ischemia, with long-term devastating complications including Volkmann ischemic contracture and limb growth disturbances. Emergency surgery within hours of birth yields good results. Badawy et al. in their case report of neonatal compartment syndrome with concomitant disseminated intravascular coagulopathy advised that the decision to perform fasciotomy in a neonate with suspected compartment syndrome should be based on a clinical diagnosis rather than compartment pressures [26].

Idiopathic spontaneous is the term for compartment syndrome that developed without any identified triggering factor. Matziolis et al. in 2012 reported the case of an otherwise healthy male treated with fasciotomies of the lower leg without any identifiable causative factor or underlying health abnormality on their extensive workout [27]. A similar case affecting the tibia was also reported by Grevitt et al. in 1991, but we must highlight that this subtype remains extremely rare in literature [28].

Other rare and atypical forms of compartment syndrome can be provoked by severe infection, and a characteristic form of that is the necrotizing fasciitis. The principles of treatment in such cases are the same with the additive effect of extensive antimicrobial treatment and extensive debridement of infected tissues. Apart from that, rare infections can cause the entity. Last year, Stull et al. reported the case of a 6-year-old man treated for compartment syndrome caused by Proteus-infected hematoma of the lower leg [29].

Vascular abnormalities such as arteriovenous malformations and fistulae can be the cause for hematoma formation and recurrent compartment syndrome. Such case was reported in the thigh of a 31-year-old fit and well male from Bournemouth who suffered ten times recurrent ACS of his thigh [30]. MR angiography at the last occurrence depicted abnormal vessels arising from profunda and superficial femoral arteries which have been embolized. This vascular abnormality was considered to arise from an old femoral fixation many years before, but the authors stated that formation during the previous fasciotomy procedures could not be excluded.

Systemic Diseases

Diabetes mellitus is considered one of the diseases making patients susceptible to developing compartment syndrome [31]. Non-enzymatic glycosylation makes diabetic collagen stiff, and microvascular alterations lead to limited joint mobility, skin alterations, and cheiroarthropathy. As a result, fascias are less distensible in potential elevation of compartmental pressures. Coley et al. in 1993 reported the case of a 44-year-old insulin-dependent diabetic woman with bilateral lower leg compartment syndrome treated effectively with fasciotomies [31]. They postulated that long-term diabetes is the cause for joint stiffness and microscopic collagen alterations. Lower and Kenzora in 1994 found that diabetic feet have elevated intramuscular compartment pressures in relation to healthy controls [32]. This mechanism in addition to diabetic collagen modulation could explain the cases of compartment syndrome reported in diabetic patients. Although it seems that long-lasting type I DM can be complicated by ACS, Flamini et al. in 2008 reported spontaneous compartment syndrome following statin administration on an asymptomatic type II diabetic patient [33]. They supported that administration of statins combined with type II DM activated a vicious circle of inflammation, edema, and necrosis.

Hypothyroidism was reported as another cause of compartment syndrome in 1993 by Thacker et al. [34]. They described bilateral lower leg ACS on a prior undiagnosed male with myxedema. In hypothyroidism, increased protein extravasation along with relatively slow lymphatic drainage leads to an increase in compartment contents [35]. On the one hand, skeletal muscle hypertrophy occurs in 1% of cases of myxoedematic myopathy [36] and is named as Hoffman's syndrome in adults and as Kocher Debre–Semelaigne syndrome in infants and children [37]. On the other hand, lack of thyroxine diminishes degradation of hyaluronate and along with TSH-derived stimulation of fibroblasts leads to increase in the connective tissues contents [38]. An increase in energy demand during mild exercise has been associated with increased risk of rhabdomyolysis in patients with uncontrolled hypothyroidism [39]. These systemic implications of hypothyroidism can explain the reported case of all-extremities compartment syndrome reported in 2016 by Musielak et al. [40]. Hypothyroidism can cause dislipidemia, which if treated with statins can both in combination cause rhabdomyolysis and concurrent ACS [41]. Therefore, in newly diagnosed dyslipidemia, screening for hypothyroidism is advocated because thyroid repletion alone can correct abnormal lipid profile and thus avoiding the risks of myopathy that statin therapy involves [42]. Primary hypothyroidism combined with adrenal insufficiency can cause rapid onset of rhabdomyolysis and myonecrosis, resulting in foot drop and poor prognosis despite treatment [43].

Hematological disorders or malignancies are known to involve or be the cause of compartment syndrome. Mostly in such cases, the underlying pathology is revealed from biopsies taken during fasciotomies for compartment syndromes of unknown origin. Non-Hodgkin lymphoma was found to infiltrate the muscles in the leg of an 80-year-old woman causing compartment syndrome, and leukemic infiltrates caused compartment syndrome in a 20-year-old man [44, 45]. In such oncological cases, aggressive tissue debridement is advised to facilitate primary closure as adjuvant chemotherapy or radiation may complicate any open wounds [46]. Myeloid sarcoma without transformation to acute myeloid leukemia (AML) has been described as a cause of ACS affecting anterior tibialis [47]. Another cause for hematological-originated ACS apart from infiltration is the excessive bleeding. Chronic phase of myeloid leukemia (CML) as a myeloproliferative disorder with excessive platelet number was found to cause ACS through excessive bleeding which persisted after fasciotomies and seized only when their number was controlled with cytosuppresive treatment [48]. However, it must be noted that in chronic CML, platelet dysfunction is not always due to their number, and urgent hematological consult should be sought [49]. Atypical ACS on grounds of chronic CML has also been described in pediatric population [50].

Clarkson reported in 1960 the first case of an otherwise fit and healthy 34-year-old Italian woman who exhibited unexplained cyclical episodes of edema and severe shock due to increase in capillary permeability which resulted in plasma shift from intravascular to the interstitial space [51]. Hemoconcentration was pronounced as red blood cells are large to be filtrated from the endothelium, and also low albumin was found. These episodes seemed to occur premenstrually, but hysterectomy and oophorectomy failed to solve the problem, and she died after a severe episode of shock. Autopsy did not shed light, and the only striking finding was monoclonal gammopathy. This rare entity was named *systemic capillary leak syndrome* (SCLS), and to date 500 cases have been described worldwide primarily in middle-aged adults [52]. It was also found to be associated with rhabdomyolysis and compartment syndrome [53]. Compartment syndrome of all four limbs has been described which was effectively treated by fasciotomies, but the syndrome itself has a poor prognosis and predisposition to multiple myeloma and leukemia [54]. SCLS presents in three phases: prodromal, extravasation, and recovery [55]. In prodromal phase, symptoms include lethargy, vomiting, abdominal pain, and generalized weakness; in extravasation phase pleuric, pericardial, epiglottic, macular, and generalized peripheral edema present along with shock; and in recovery phase, pulmonary edema can occur due to the mobilization of fluid to intravascular space. It is important not to overlook other usual cases of shock and allergies. The etiology of this syndrome remains unknown, no familiar distribution was found, and various treatments such as theophyllines, terbutaline, steroids, plasmapheresis and thalidomide have been employed with variable success, leaving a mortality rate of 25–30%. In June of this year, the first metanalysis of published SCLS in childhood depicted 24 relevant studies and showed that the syndrome also affects childhood and follows acute illness in 75% but not related to any monoclonal gammopathy [56].

Human immunodeficiency virus (HIV) infection can also rarely be complicated by compartment syndrome. The pathophysiology may vary: HIV-induced thrombocytopenia causing bleeding and myositis from antiretroviral treatment have been reported [57, 58]. A rare case of bilateral spontaneous lower leg compartment syndrome was attributed to antiretroviral-induced myositis [59].

Moreover, compartment syndrome of the hand has been reported in a case of *multiple sclerosis* possibly associated with the cutaneous changes of that syndrome [60].

Drugs

Statins (hydroxymethylglutaryl coenzyme A (HMG-CoA) reductase inhibitors are widely prescribed to treat hyperlipidemia. Myogenic damage is known to be one of their side effects. Coadministration of simvastastion with risperidone (atypical neuroleptic drug) has been reported as a cause of compartment syndrome [61]. It was postulated that risperidone may have diminished the metabolism of simvastatin via interactions with the cytochrome P450 (CYP) system, resulting in marked plasma elevation of simvastatin and consequent rhabdomyolysis and compartment syndrome.

Serotonin syndrome was also reported as a cause of compartment syndrome [62]. This syndrome involves encephalopathy, neuromuscular contractures, and clonus and autonomic hyperactivity. A 68-year-old woman was taking paroxetine (a selective serotonin reuptake inhibitor (SSRI)) and risperidone and sustained a serotonin syndrome with consequent rhabdomyolysis and compartment syndrome of both legs. As a causative factor, the serotonin syndrome was suspected, but coadministration of risperidone may have played its role. Risperidone was also found to be the cause of bilateral tibial compartment syndrome in a 31-year-old man suffering from schizophrenia after 1 and half hours of walking without any other predisposing factors [63].

Lithium has also been reported as causing an atypical form of compartment syndrome: atraumatic, painless, and affecting only one out of four tibial compartments [64]. It is considered as pain-perception altering with effect to pain receptors so patients appear obtunded.

Unusual Anatomical Locations

Gluteal compartment syndrome is rare. Gluteal compartments were described in the cadaveric study of David et al.: three compartments from lateral to medial with one enclosing tensor fascia lata, one gluteus medius plus minimus, and one containing gluteus maximus [65]. Sciatic nerve dysfunction is a common clinical finding in gluteal compartment syndrome despite the fact that sciatic nerve is enclosed within a separate compartment. Sciatic involvement is mostly attributed to external compression on its arterial supply, which most commonly arises from the medial circumflex femoral and inferior gluteal arteries. Out of the two branches of the sciatic nerve, the peroneal (fibular) is more susceptible to injury; thus, the patients may present with only isolated foot drop [66]. The nonspecific symptoms of buttock swelling and tenderness often lead to misdiagnosis such as pelvic or lower limb venous thrombosis, and the initiated antithrombotic treatment further aggravates any gluteal hematomas, resulting in even higher compartmental pressures [67]. Differentiation between gluteal compartment syndrome and thrombosis requires CPK measurement, intracompartmental pressure measurement, and imaging studies. No definition of the threshold of abnormal raised intracompartmental pressure is needed to diagnose gluteal compartment syndrome. Normal values have been reported to be 13–14 mm Hg [68]. Emergent fasciotomies are considered the treatment of choice, and even in delayed presentation after 56 hours, they provided a favorable outcome [69]. Therefore, Panagiotopoulos et al. on their case report with residual sciatic nerve palsy despite fasciotomies reported that nonoperative treatment should have limited place due to high risks and minimal benefits [66]. Kocher-Langenbeck approach is usually used for the gluteal fasciotomies. Henson et al. in 2009 published the first and only systematic review of gluteal compartment syndrome [70]. They reviewed seven papers (28 cases) which were all retrospective case reports and summarized that the causes of compartment syndrome affecting the gluteal region can be trauma, vascular injury or surgery, intramuscular drug abuse, altered level of consciousness from alcohol intake or drug overdose, prolonged immobilization, epidural anesthesia after joint arthroplasty, and infection. On their systematic review, half of the papers had prolonged immobilization as the leading cause. Diagnosis was based solely on clinical symptoms in 53.6%, and intracompartmental pressures greater than 30 mmHg were considered as definite indication for surgical treatment. Surgical fasciotomies were the preferred method of treatment in 71.4% of the cases, and only 12 out of 25 cases recovered fully. Therefore, authors highlighted that gluteal compartment syndrome implies a big cause of patient disability and that there is a lack of an adopted system of precise indications for surgery and of functional evaluation regardless of the way of treatment. Gluteal compartment syndrome has been reported as a complication after bone marrow biopsy from iliac crest to a patient who was anticoagulated [71]. The same complication was reported after posterior iliac crest marrow biopsy of a patient suffering from non-Hodgkin lymphoma; however, on this case, platelet number and clotting times were normal [72].

Compartment syndrome in lumbar region may be a cause of severe low back pain according to Peck in 1981 [73]. Lumbar paraspinal compartment syndrome was then officially described in 1985 by Carr in a young man with severe low back pain after exertion [74]. It seems that recently weight lifting including "CrossFit," which have gained popularity, have accounted for many of such compartment cases reported. Paraspinal muscles are enclosed by the thoracolumbar fascia which behaves like a closed space with resting intracompartmental pressures varying from 3 to 7.95 mmHg, depending on the position and being elevated up to 25 mmHg during exercise [75]. Patients present typically with severe low back pain, bilateral symptoms, swollen paraspinal muscles, pain in the hip flexion but not in straight leg raise, and absent bowel sounds due to ileus. Diagnostic modalities such as MRI or CT, though not used routinely in compartment syndrome of extremities, play a significant role in diagnosis of lumbar paraspinal compartment syndrome. Paramedian Wiltse incision rather than a midline is used as it allows for delayed soft tissue closure or grafting over a viable muscle bed [76]. After the release of the fascia, the relevant compartments of longissimus, iliocostalis, spinalis, and multifidus are approached. Alexander et al. this year published the first systematic review of acute paraspinal compartment syndrome [77]. They assessed 21 retrospective case reports and found that the cause was mainly not related to direct trauma to spinal muscles but in 52 % of cases was related to weightlifting and the rest to other sport activities such as skiing or surfing and spinal surgery. Intracompartmental pressures were measured with patient prone and averaged to 73.7 mmHg, much higher than other body locations. Fasciotomies were applied in twelve of the twenty-one case reports, where nine of them received medical treatment and two hyperbaric oxygen therapy. All cases treated surgically even with delays up to 7 days had a good outcome, whereas all conservative and hyperbaric oxygen cases had ongoing symptoms or functional deficit. Therefore, they suggested that surgical decompression on confirmed diagnosis should be the treatment of choice regardless of the delay of diagnosis. Only one case of chronic lumbar paraspinal compartment syndrome is reported after weight lifting and was treated successfully with bilateral minimally invasive fasciotomies at L3 level under local anesthesia [78]. Fascia was found thickened, and samples confirmed the hyperplastic muscle fibers. The patient after 4 weeks returned to his weight lifting training for the 2008 Olympics without any residual symptoms.

Other unusual anatomical locations which can be affected by compartment syndrome are the medial head of gastrocnemius (tennis leg) and peroneus longus [79, 80].

Procedures

Coronary artery bypass grafting can be complicated by leg compartment syndrome [81]. The exact mechanism is unknown, although prolonged bypass time or saphenous vein harvesting on patients under statins has been implicated as risk factors.

Total knee replacements in very rare occasions have been associated with compartment syndrome of either the glutei, thigh, or tibia. As regards the tibia, this situation cannot be explained as the replacement takes place in a different compartment [82]. However, tourniquet time, epidural anesthesia, continuous passive movement device, thromboprophylaxis, and aggressive physiotherapy have all been thought as contributing factors without a clear correlation being identified with the exception of the tourniquet time. Functional outcomes after fasciotomies remain moderate mainly due to periprosthetic infections.

Postprocedural compartment syndrome resulting from placement of neuromonitoring needles in forearm has also been described [83]. Patients undergoing such endovascular procedures are on antiplatelet treatment, and therefore at an increased risk of bleeding and elevated intracompartmental pressures. Prevention can be achieved by extra vigilance to avoid superficial veins and vertical insertion to the skin.

Unusual Fractures

Innocuous distal radius in elderly and low demand patients have been reported to be complicated by compartment syndrome. This was an extremely rare manifestation unable to be explained by fracture displacement, mechanism, and severity of injury or any other factors. In one case, amputation of digits was performed despite initial fasciotomy [84]. Chloros et al. in their paper highlighted the significance of the pronator quadratus space and its potential role [85].

Take-Home Message
- Compartment syndrome can present atypically and in variable context. Raised awareness on a suspected case can prove limb/lifesaving.
- Systemic diseases, drugs, rare body locations, unusual conditions and fractures, and common surgical procedures can all be associated with this syndrome.
- Symptoms do not differ from a usual acute compartment syndrome.
- Measurement of intracompartmental pressures should not delay treatment in highly suspicious cases with clear clinical symptoms.
- Irrespective of the cause, condition, or location, surgical fasciotomies of involved compartments remain the treatment of choice as per acute compartment syndrome (ACS).
- Due to their atypical manifestation, delays in treatment can commonly appear unfavoring its final prognosis.

References

1. Robinson MS, Parekh AA, Smith WR, et al. Bilateral exercise induced exertional compartment syndrome resulting in acute compartment loss: a case report. J Trauma. 2008;65:225–7.
2. Edwards P, Myerson MS. Exertional compartment syndrome of the leg. Phys Sports Med. 1996;24(4)
3. Edmundsson D, Toolanen G, Sojka P. Chronic compartment syndrome also affects nonathletic subjects. A prospective study of 63 cases with exercise-induced lower leg pain. Acta Orthop. 2007;78(1):136–42.
4. Livingston KS, Meehan WP, Hresko MT, Matheney TH, Shore BJ. Acute exertional compartment syndrome in young athletes: a descriptive case series and review of the literature. Pediatr Emerg Care. 2018;34(2):76–80. https://doi.org/10.1097/PEC.0000000000000647.
5. Chan RK, Austen WG Jr, Ibrahim S, et al. Reperfusion injury to skeletal muscle affects primarily type II muscle fibers. J Surg Res. 2004;122:54–60.
6. McKinney B, Gaunder C, Schumer R. Acute exertional compartment syndrome with rhabdomyolysis: case report and review of literature. Am J Case Rep. 2018;19:145–9.
7. Nicholson P, Devitt A, Stevens M, Mahalingum K. Acute exertional peroneal compartmental syndrome following prolonged horse riding. Injury. 1998;29(8):643–4.
8. Sit YK, Lui TH. Acute compartment syndrome after medial gastrocnemius tear. Foot Ankle Spec. 2015;8(1):65–7. https://doi.org/10.1177/1938640014543360. Epub 2014 Jul 21.
9. Bunting L, Briggs B. An unusual complication of weightlifting: a case report. Ann Emerg Med. 2014;63(3):357–60. https://doi.org/10.1016/j.annemergmed.2013.05.005. Epub 2013 Jun 28.
10. Irion V, Magnussen RA, Miller TL, Kaeding CC. Return to activity following fasciotomy for chronic exertional compartment syndrome. Eur J Orthop Surg Traumatol. 2014;24(7):1223–8. https://doi.org/10.1007/s00590-014-1433-0. Epub 2014 Mar 25.
11. Clanton TO, Solcher BW. Chronic leg pain in the athlete. Clin Sports Med. 1994;13:743–59.
12. Shah SN, Miller BS, Kuhn JE. Chronic exertional compartment syndrome. Am J Orthop (Belle Mead NJ). 2004;33:335–41.
13. Tucker AK. Chronic exertional compartment syndrome of the leg. Curr Rev Musculoskelet Med. 2010;3:32–7.

14. Tzortziou V, Maffulli N, Padhiar N. Diagnosis and management of chronic exertional compartment syndrome (CECS) in the United Kingdom. Clin J Sport Med. 2006;16:209–13.
15. Rorabeck CH, Bourne RB, Fowler PJ, Finlay JB, Nott L. The role of tissue pressure measurement in diagnosing chronic anterior compartment syndrome. Am J Sports Med. 1988;16: 143–6.
16. Pedowitz RA, Hargens AR, Mubarak SJ, Gershuni DH. Modified criteria for the objective diagnosis of chronic compartment syndrome of the leg. Am J Sports Med. 1990;18(1): 35–40.
17. Roberts A, Franklyn-Miller A. The validity of the diagnostic criteria used in chronic exertional compartment syndrome: a systematic review. Scand J Med Sci Sports. 2012;22(5):585–95. https://doi.org/10.1111/j.1600-0838.2011.01386.x. Epub 2011 Sep 13.
18. Brennan FH Jr, Kane SF. Diagnosis, treatment options, and rehabilitation of chronic lower leg exertional compartment syndrome. Curr Sports Med Rep. 2003;2:247–50.
19. Detmer DE, Sharpe K, Sufit RL, Girdley FM. Chronic compartment syndrome: diagnosis, management, and outcomes. Am J Sports Med. 1985;13:162–70.
20. Pozzi A, Pivato G, Kask K, Susini F, Pegoli L. Single portal endoscopic treatment for chronic exertional compartment syndrome of the forearm. Tech Hand Up Extreme Surg. 2014;18(3):153–6. https://doi.org/10.1097/BTH.0000000000000056.
21. Ragland R 3rd, Moukoko D, Ezaki M, et al. Forearm compartment syndrome in the newborn: report of 24 cases. J Hand Surg. 2005;30:997–1003.
22. Goubier JN, Romaña C, Molina V. Neonatal Volkmann's compartment syndrome: a report of two cases. Chir Main. 2005;24(1):45–7.
23. Plancq MC, Buisson P, Deroussen F, Krim G, Collet LM, Gouron R. Successful early surgical treatment in neonatal compartment syndrome: case report. J Hand Surg Am. 2013;38(6):1185–8. https://doi.org/10.1016/j.jhsa.2013.03.029. Epub 2013 May 9.
24. Hensinger RN. Gangrene of the newborn: a case report. J Bone Joint Surg Am. 1975;57(1):121–3.
25. Léauté-Labrèze C, Depaire-Duclos F, Sarlangue J, et al. Congenital cutaneous defects as complications in surviving co-twins: aplasia cutis congenital and neonatal volkmann ischemic contracture of the forearm. Arch Dermatol. 1998;134(9):1121–4.
26. Badawy SM, Gust MJ, Liem RI, Ball MK, Gosain AK, Sharathkumar AA. Neonatal compartment syndrome associated with disseminated intravascular coagulation. Ann Plast Surg. 2016;76(2):256–8. https://doi.org/10.1097/SAP.0000000000000522.
27. Matziolis G, Erli HJ, Rau MH, Klever P, Paar O. Idiopathic compartment syndrome: a case report. J Trauma. 2002;53(1):122–4.
28. Grevitt MP, Macdonald RF. Spontaneous tibial compartment syndrome. Injury. 1991;22(4):330.
29. Stull J, Bhat S, Miller AJ, Hoffman R, Wang ML. Treatment of atypical compartment syndrome due to proteus infection. Orthopedics. 2017;40(1):e176–8. https://doi.org/10.3928/01477447-20160926-08. Epub 2016 Sep 30.
30. Rohman L, Chan S, Hadi S, Maruszewski D. Recurrent spontaneous compartment syndrome of the thigh. BMJ Case Rep. 2014;2014. pii: bcr2013201859. https://doi.org/10.1136/bcr-2013-201859.
31. Coley S, Situnayake RD, Allen MJ. Compartment syndrome, stiff joints, and diabetic cheiroarthropathy. Ann Rheum Dis. 1993;52(11):840.
32. Lower RF, Kenzora JE. The diabetic neuropathic foot: a triple crush syndrome-measurement of compartmental pressures of normal and diabetic feet. Orthopedics. 1994;17(3):241–8.
33. Flamini S, Zoccali C, Persi E, Calvisi V. Spontaneous compartment syndrome in a patient with diabetes and statin administration: a case report. J Orthop Traumatol. 2008;9(2):101–3. https://doi.org/10.1007/s10195-008-0004-8. Epub 2008 May 14.
34. Thacker AK, Agrawal D, Sarkari NB. Bilateral anterior tibial compartment syndrome in association with hypothyroidism. Postgrad Med J. 1993;69(817):881–3.
35. Parving H, Hansen JM, Nilsen SV, Rossing N, Munck O, Lassen NA. Mechanisms of edema formation in myxedema - increased protein extra-vasation and relatively slow lymphatic drainage. N Engl J Med. 1981;301:460.

36. Ramsay ID. Endocrine myopathies. Practitioner. 1982;226:1075–80.
37. Klein I, Parker M, Shebert R, et al. Hypothyroidism presenting as muscle stiffness and pseudo-hypertrophy: Hoffman's syndrome. Am J Med. 1981;70:891–4.
38. Bland JH, Frymoyer JW. Rheumatic syndromes of myxedema. N Engl J Med. 1970;282(21):1171–4.
39. Riggs JE. Acute exertional rhabdomyolysis in hypothyroidism: the result of a reversible defect in glycogenolysis. Mil Med. 1990;155:171–2.
40. Musielak MC, Chae JH. Hypothyroid-induced acute compartment syndrome in all extremities. J Surg Case Rep. 2016;2016(12) https://doi.org/10.1093/jscr/rjw215. pii: rjw215.
41. Chaudhary N, Duggal AK, Makhija P, Puri V, Khwaja GA. Statin-induced bilateral foot drop in a case of hypothyroidism. Ann Indian Acad Neurol. 2015;18(3):331–4. https://doi.org/10.4103/0972-2327.157251.
42. Ladenson PW, Singer PA, Ain KB, Bagchi N, Bigos ST, Levy EG, et al. American thyroid association guidelines for detection of thyroid dysfunction. Arch Intern Med. 2000;160:1573–5.
43. Muir P, Choe MS, Croxson MS. Rapid development of anterotibial compartment syndrome and rhabdomyolysis in a patient with primary hypothyroidism and adrenal insufficiency. Thyroid. 2012;22(6):651–3. https://doi.org/10.1089/thy.2011.0136. Epub 2012 May 8.
44. Southworth SR, O'Malley NP, Ebraheim NA, Zeff L, Cummings V. Compartment syndrome as a presentation of non-Hodgkin's lymphoma. J Orthop Trauma. 1990;4(4):470–3.
45. Trumble T. Forearm compartment syndrome secondary to leukemic infiltrates. J Hand Surg Am. 1987;12(4):563–5.
46. Veeragandham RS, Paz IB, Nadeemanee A. Compartment syndrome of the leg secondary to leukemic infiltration: a case report and review of the literature. J Surg Oncol. 1994;55(3):198–200; discussion 200-1.
47. Scheipl S, Leithner A, Radl R, Beham-Schmid C, Ranner G, Linkesch W, Windhager R. Myeloid sarcoma presenting in muscle-tissue of the lower limb: unusual origin of a compartment-syndrome. Am J Clin Oncol. 2007;30(6):658–9.
48. Nagase Y, Ueda S, Matsunaga H, et al. Acute compartment syndrome as the initial manifestation of chronic-phase chronic myeloid leukemia: a case report and review of the literature. J Med Case Rep. 2016;10:201. https://doi.org/10.1186/s13256-016-0985-5.
49. Ng AP, Servadei P, Tuckfield A, Friedhuber A, Grigg A. Resolution of platelet function defects with imatinib therapy in a patient with chronic myeloid leukaemia in chronic phase. Blood Coagul Fibrinolysis. 2009;20(1):81–3. https://doi.org/10.1097/MBC.0b013e3283177b03.
50. Cohen E, Truntzer J, Klinge S, Schwartz K, Schiller J. Acute pediatric leg compartment syndrome in chronic myeloid leukemia. Orthopedics. 2014;37(11):e1036–9. https://doi.org/10.3928/01477447-20141023-91.
51. Clarkson B, Thompson D, Horwith M, Luckey EH. Cyclical edema and shock due to increased capillary permeability. Trans Assoc Am Phys. 1960;73:272–82.
52. Siddall E, Khatri M, Radhakrishnan J. Capillary leak syndrome: etiologies, pathophysiology, and management. Kidney Int. 2017;92(1):37–46. https://doi.org/10.1016/j.kint.2016.11.029.
53. Prieto Valderrey F, Burillo Putze G, Martinez Azario J, Santana Ramos M. Systemic capillary leak syndrome associated with rhabdomyolysis and compartment syndrome. Am J Emerg Med. 1999;17(7):743–4.
54. Milner CS, Wagstaff MJ, Rose GK. Compartment syndrome of multiple limbs: an unusual presentation. J Plast Reconstr Aesthet Surg. 2006;59(11):1251–2. Epub 2006 Jun 6.
55. Kyeremanteng K, D'Egidio G, Wan C, Baxter A, Rosenberg H. Compartment syndrome as a result of systemic capillary leak syndrome. Case Rep Crit Care. 2016;2016:4206397. https://doi.org/10.1155/2016/4206397. Epub 2016 Sep 5.
56. Bozzini MA, Milani GP, Bianchetti MG, Fossali EF, Lava SAG. Idiopathic systemic capillary leak syndrome (Clarkson syndrome) in childhood: systematic literature review. Eur J Pediatr 2018. https://doi.org/10.1007/s00431-018-3189-8. [Epub ahead of print].

57. Desai SS, McCarthy CK, Kestin A, et al. Acute forearm compartment syndrome associated with HIV-induced thrombocytopenia. J Hand Surg Am. 1993;18:865–7.
58. Lam R, Lin PH, Alankar S, et al. Acute limb ischemia secondary to myositis-induced compartment syndrome in a patient with human immunodeficiency virus infection. J Vasc Surg. 2003;37:1103–5.
59. Davidson DJ, Shaukat YM, Jenabzadeh R, Gupte CM. Spontaneous bilateral compartment syndrome in a HIV-positive patient. BMJ Case Rep. 2013;2013. pii: bcr-2013-202651. https://doi.org/10.1136/bcr-2013-202651.
60. Tanagho A, Hatab S, Youssef S, Ansara S. Spontaneous compartment syndrome of the hand in systemic sclerosis. Orthopedics. 2015;38(9):e849–51. https://doi.org/10.3928/01477447-20150902-91.
61. Webber MA, Mahmud W, Lightfoot JD, Shekhar A. Rhabdomyolysis and compartment syndrome with coadministration of risperidone and simvastatin. J Psychopharmacol. 2004;18(3):432–4.
62. Clarissa Samara V, Warner J. Rare case of severe serotonin syndrome leading to bilateral compartment syndrome. BMJ Case Rep. 2017;2017. pii: bcr2016218842. https://doi.org/10.1136/bcr-2016-218842.
63. Rochcongar G, Maigné G, Pineau V, Hulet C. Walking and risperidone: a rare cause of acute compartment syndrome. Joint Bone Spine. 2013;80(5):542–3. https://doi.org/10.1016/j.jbspin.2013.02.006. Epub 2013 Apr 6.
64. Oh LS, Lewis PB, Prasarn ML, Lorich DG, Helfet DL. Painless, atraumatic, isolated lateral compartment syndrome of the leg: an unusual triad of atypical findings. Am J Orthop (Belle Mead NJ). 2010;39(1):35–9.
65. David V, Thambiah J, Kagda FH, Kumar VP. Bilateral gluteal compartment syndrome. A case report. J Bone Joint Surg Am. 2005;87(11):2541–5.
66. Panagiotopoulos AC, Vrachnis I, Kraniotis P, Tyllianakis M. Gluteal compartment syndrome following drug-induced immobilization: a case report. BMC Res Notes. 2015;8:35. https://doi.org/10.1186/s13104-015-1003-5.
67. Taylor BC, Dimitris C, Tancevski A, Tran JL. Gluteal compartment syndrome and superior gluteal artery injury as a result of simple hip dislocation: a case report. Iowa Orthop J. 2011;31:181–6.
68. Yoshioka H. Gluteal compartment syndrome. A report of 4 cases. Acta Orthop Scand. 1992;63:347–9.
69. Lawrence JE, Cundall-Curry DJ, Stohr KK. Delayed presentation of gluteal compartment syndrome: the argument for fasciotomy. Case Rep Orthop. 2016;2016:9127070. https://doi.org/10.1155/2016/9127070. Epub 2016 Mar 17.
70. Henson JT, Roberts CS, Giannoudis PV. Gluteal compartment syndrome. Acta Orthop Belg. 2009;75:147–52.
71. McGoldrick NP, Green C, Connolly P. Gluteal compartment syndrome following bone marrow biopsy: a case report. Acta Orthop Belg. 2012;78:548–51.
72. Berumen-Nafarrate E, Vega-Najera C, Leal-Contreras C, Leal-Berumen I. Gluteal compartment syndrome following an iliac bone marrow aspiration. Case Rep Orthop. 2013;2013:812172. https://doi.org/10.1155/2013/812172. Epub 2013 Dec 11.
73. Peck D. Evidence for the existence of compartment syndrome of the epaxial muscles. Anat Rec. 1981;198:199–201.
74. Carr D, Gilbertson L, Frymoyer J, Krag M, Pope M. Lumbar paraspinal compartment syndrome. A case report with physiologic and anatomic studies. Spine (Phila Pa 1976). 1985;10(9):816–20.
75. Songcharoen P, Chotigavanich C, Thanapipatsiri S. Lumbar paraspinal compartment pressure in back muscle exercise. J Spinal Disord. 1994;7:49–53.
76. Wiltse LL, Bateman JG, Hutchinson RH, Nelson WE. The paraspinal sacrospinalis splitting approach to the lumbar spine. J Bone Joint Surg Am. 1968;50(5):919–26.

77. Alexander W, Low N, Pratt G. Acute lumbar paraspinal compartment syndrome: a systematic review. ANZ J Surg. 2018; https://doi.org/10.1111/ans.14342. [Epub ahead of print].
78. Xu YM, Bai YH, Li QT, Yu H, Cao ML. Chronic lumbar paraspinal compartment syndrome: a case report and review of the literature. J Bone Joint Surg Br. 2009;91(12):1628–30. https://doi.org/10.1302/0301-620X.91B12.22647.
79. Tao L, Jun H, Muliang D, Deye S, Jiangdong N. Acute compartment syndrome after gastrocnemius rupture (tennis leg) in a nonathlete without trauma. J Foot Ankle Surg. 2016;55(2):303–5. https://doi.org/10.1053/j.jfas.2014.09.022. Epub 2014 Nov 27.
80. Merriman J, Villacis D, Kephart C, Yi A, Romano R, Hatch GF 3rd. Acute compartment syndrome after non-contact peroneus longus muscle rupture. Clin Orthop Surg. 2015;7(4):527–30. https://doi.org/10.4055/cios.2015.7.4.527. Epub 2015 Nov 13.
81. Etra JW, Metkus TS, Whitman GJ, Mandal K. Lower extremity compartment syndrome after coronary artery bypass: easy to miss unless suspected. Ann Thorac Surg. 2016;101(1):e13–4. https://doi.org/10.1016/j.athoracsur.2015.06.110.
82. Shaath M, Sukeik M, Mortada S, Masterson S. Compartment syndrome following total knee replacement: a case report and literature review. World J Orthop. 2016;(7, 9):618–22. https://doi.org/10.5312/wjo.v7.i9.618. eCollection 2016 Sep 18.
83. Eli IM, Gamboa NT, Guan J, Taussky P. Acute compartment syndrome as a complication of the use of intraoperative neuromonitoring needle electrodes. World Neurosurg. 2018;112:247–9. https://doi.org/10.1016/j.wneu.2018.01.192. Epub 2018 Feb 3.
84. Egro FM, Jaring MR, Khan AZ. Compartment syndrome of the hand: beware of innocuous radius fractures. Eplasty. 2014;14:e6. eCollection 2014.
85. Chloros GD, Papadonikolakis A, Ginn S, Wiesler ER. Pronator quadratus space and compartment syndrome after low-energy fracture of the distal radius: a case report. J Surg Orthop Adv. 2008 Summer;17(2):102–6.

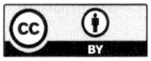

Chapter 16
Common Misperceptions Among Health-Care Professionals

Joshua A. Parry

Background to the Problem

- Misperceptions regarding the causes, presentation, and diagnosis of acute compartment syndrome (ACS) can lead to a delay in its diagnosis and treatment that negatively impact patient outcomes.
- The misperceptions, low incidence, and numerous causes of acute compartment syndrome result in a low level of awareness among health-care professionals.
- There is controversy surrounding the best method to diagnose acute compartment syndrome.
- A high degree of suspicion among health-care professionals is necessary to prevent a delay in the diagnosis of acute compartment syndrome.

What Is Recommended

Misperceptions regarding the causes, presentation, and diagnosis of acute compartment syndrome (ACS) can lead to a delay in its diagnosis and treatment that negatively impact patient outcomes. Health-care professionals should be properly educated on ACS to dispel these misperceptions in order to prevent the devastating consequences of a missed compartment syndrome.

Misperception #1: Open fractures do not develop acute compartment syndrome

Up to 70% of ACS occurs in the presence of fractures, most commonly the tibial shaft (36%) and the distal radius (10%) [1]. Open fractures present with a defect in the fascial compartments and might intuitively thought to be at a lower risk of ACS

J. A. Parry (✉)
Denver Health Medical Center, Department of Orthopedics, Denver, CO, USA

© The Author(s) 2019
C. Mauffrey et al. (eds.), *Compartment Syndrome*,
https://doi.org/10.1007/978-3-030-22331-1_16

Fig. 16.1 Photograph of a patient presenting with a grossly open femur fracture who subsequently developed acute compartment syndrome. Large open wounds do not preclude the development of acute compartment syndrome

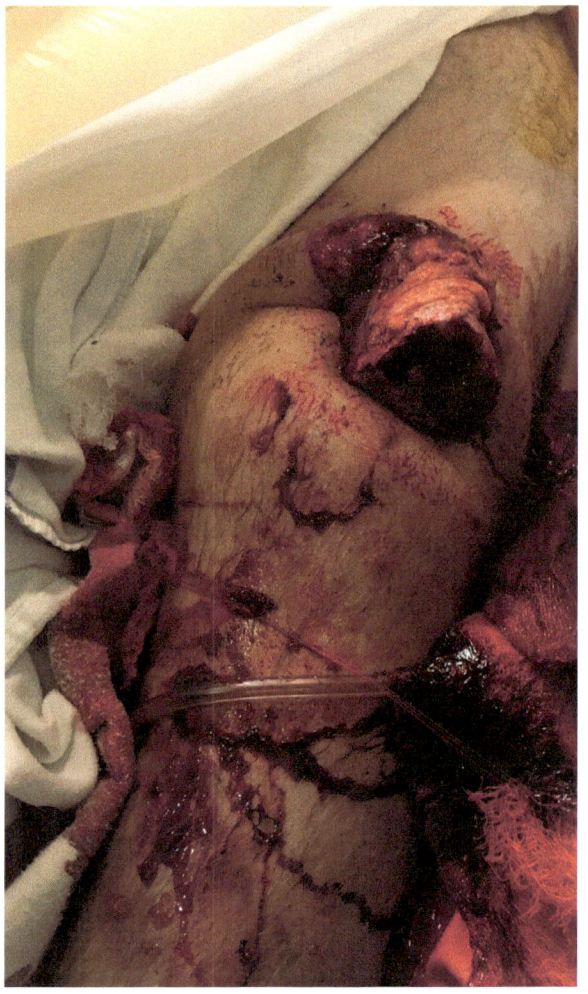

(Fig. 16.1). However, the incidence of ACS in open tibial shaft fractures has not been shown to differ from that of closed fractures, ranging from 5% to 9%, with all four compartments of the leg being susceptible to ACS [2–4]. Providers must continue to monitor these patients for the signs and symptoms of ACS in the setting of open fracture.

Misperception #2: A diagnosis of acute compartment syndrome is unlikely if there is no fracture

Around 30% of all ACS presents without an associated fracture [5]. When ACS presents without a fracture, a delayed diagnosis is more likely [1, 5]. Hope et al. [5] found a significantly longer delay to fasciotomy for ACS without fracture (34 versus 21 hours) along with a higher incidence of muscle necrosis at the time of fasciotomy (21% vs 8%) suggesting that this delay was detrimental to the patient.

There are numerous causes of ACS that do not involve fracture, including both traumatic and nontraumatic causes [6, 7]. Traumatic causes include injuries that crush, burn, penetrate, or compress. Even minor trauma can result in ACS in patients with bleeding disorders or anticoagulation medication. Nontraumatic causes include, but are not limited to, ischemia–reperfusion injuries, bleeding diatheses, intravenous (IV) extravasation, IV drug abuse, envenomation, nephrotic syndrome, and infection. The extensive list of potential causes means that ACS can present to health-care professionals over a wide range of specialties making it necessary for all providers to understand the presentation and diagnosis of ACS in order to prevent a delay in its treatment.

Misperception #3: The five "Ps" of acute compartment syndrome: Pain, pallor, pulselessness, parasthesias, and paralysis
It is important to consider ACS in the setting of any painful and tense muscle compartment. It has been classically taught that the clinical exam findings of ACS present as the "5 Ps" (pain, pallor, pulselessness, paresthesias, and paralysis) [3, 6, 7]. However, these findings represent arterial insufficiency and typically present in the late stages of compartment syndrome [6, 8, 9]. Instead, the "5 Ps" of ACS have been recommended by one author to be changed to pain, pain, pain, pain, and more pain; specifically, pain with passive stretch of the muscle compartment, pain out of proportion to that of the injury, and pain that is unresponsive to adequate analgesia [6]. Despite this recommendation, the sensitivity of pain is still low [9]. An analysis of four prospective trials involving the lower extremity determined that pain, pain with passive stretch, and paresthesias on exam had a sensitivity of 13–19% and a specificity of 97–98%, suggesting that the absence of these symptoms was better at excluding the diagnosis than ruling it in [9]. The presence of multiple clinical findings does increase the probability, with the likelihood of ACS increasing from 25%, to 68%, and to 98% with one, two, and three findings, respectively. Additionally, the ability of physicians to discern critically high intracompartmental pressure from baseline levels via palpation of muscle compartments has been shown to be poor and should not be relied on [10].

Misperception #4: A one-time elevated intracompartmental pressure measurement is diagnostic of acute compartment syndrome
There is no clear validated criteria for when ACS is actually present [7]. There is controversy surrounding the appropriate method to diagnose ACS. Classically, ACS has been diagnosed by the clinical exam of an awake and alert patient, while ICP monitoring is reserved for those with unreliable clinical exams. This is reflected in a recent survey of orthopedic traumatologists that demonstrated a strong consensus that the diagnosis of ACS should be made clinically based on the presence of a tense muscle compartment, pain with passive stretch, and pain out of proportion to the injury [11]. There was also a strong consensus that ICP monitoring should be used when the clinical exam was unreliable such as in children, multiply injured, or obtunded patients. In contrast, the routine use ICP monitoring in awake and alert patients was only supported by 18% of the respondents. While the clinical exam may be the standard for diagnosing ACS for many, the poor sensitivity of these

findings has led some authors to recommend for routine ICP monitoring in at-risk patients [1, 7, 12]. Mcqueen et al. [13] were able to correctly identify all cases of ACS in a prospective cohort using a perfusion differential threshold of less than 30 mmHg between the diastolic blood pressure and the ICP. While this method is highly sensitive resulting in very few missed cases of ACS, other authors argue that ICP monitoring is not only costly and burdensome for the hospital staff but also nonspecific, leading to gross overtreatment [14, 15]. This appears to be especially true if one-time ICP measurements are used to make the diagnosis [14–16]. Whitney et al. [14] performed one-time ICP measurements in tibial shaft fractures with no exam findings of ACS and found that 35% of patients had perfusion differential <30 mmHg demonstrating that the use of this threshold would have led to a high rate of unnecessary fasciotomies in this population. In contrast to one-time ICP measurements, Mcqueen et al. [12] reviewed 850 tibial shaft fractures that under-went routine continuous ICP monitoring and found that a mean perfusion differen-tial threshold of less than 30 mmHg for two consecutive hours had excellent sensitivity and specificity, 94% and 98%, respectively, for diagnosing ACS, making a strong argument for the use of routine continuous ICP monitoring in at-risk patients.

Limitations and Pitfalls

The misperceptions of ACS can ultimately result in a delayed or missed diagnosis, both of which can be devastating for patients. The timely and accurate diagnosis of ACS remains challenging due to the multitude of insults that can cause it, the incon-sistent exam findings, and its presence in patients who cannot reliably communi-cate. These difficulties make a delayed diagnosis of ACS nearly inevitable. Physicians, advanced practitioners, and nurses must be appropriately educated to dispel the abovementioned misperceptions in order to have the appropriate level of suspicion necessary to detect and treat ACS in a timely manner. Whether using clinical exam findings, ICP monitoring, or both to diagnose ACS, it is important to understand that ACS is a disease process that develops over time making serial examinations or continuous ICP monitoring a necessity.

Future Directions

Continued education and institutional protocols are potential tools for correcting the misperceptions of ACS. In an effort to improve the early identification of ACS at one academic hospital, Schaffzin et al. [17] implemented a series of changes with the goal of increasing the number of at-risk patients that received appropriate orders for, performance of, and documentation of serial neurovascular examinations. These institutional changes included provider and nursing reminders, modifications to electronic medical record order sets, mandatory education, and formal lectures. The use of chart inserts and checklists have also been used to help increase the identification and monitoring of at-risk patients for ACS [18].

The implementation of educational programs, order sets, and checklists may be able to better identify and monitor patients at risk of ACS; however, additional research is still necessary to develop clear and validated criteria for when ACS is actually present. Advanced diagnostic tests for the identification of ACS have been investigated extensively, including biomarkers for muscle damage and ischemia, magnetic resonance imaging, ultrasound, scintigraphy, laser Doppler flowmetry, near-infrared spectroscopy, and direct hardness measurements, but none of these tests have demonstrated superiority to the clinical exam and ICP monitoring [3, 7]. Schimdt et al. [19] performed a multicenter prospective trial that combined continuous ICP monitoring, near-infrared spectroscopy muscle oxygenation, clinical exam findings, and 6-month outcome scores in order to develop a predictive model for ACS. The application of this predictive model to future prospective studies has the potential to develop a more reliable diagnostic criteria for ACS.

Take-Home Message
- Acute compartment syndrome should be considered in at-risk patients presenting with a tense painful muscle compartment.
- Open fractures are still at risk of developing acute compartment syndrome.
- Acute compartment syndrome presenting without a fracture is more likely to have a delayed diagnosis.
- Pain is the only reliable early clinical finding, while pallor, pulselessness, paresthesias, and paralysis present later.
- Reliance on one-time intracompartmental pressure monitoring will result in a high rate of unnecessary fasciotomies.
- Continuous intracompartmental pressure monitoring is the most sensitive and specific test for acute compartment syndrome.
- Educational programs, order sets, checklists, and improved diagnostic techniques are potential tools to dispel the misperceptions of acute compartment syndrome and to prevent a delayed diagnosis.

References

1. McQueen MM, Gaston P, Court-Brown CM. Acute compartment syndrome. Who is at risk? J Bone Joint Surg Br [Internet]. 2000 Mar [cited 2018 Apr 8];82(2):200–3. Available from: http://www.ncbi.nlm.nih.gov/pubmed/10755426.
2. Blick SS, Brumback RJ, Poka A, et al. Compartment syndrome in open tibial fractures. J Bone Joint Surg Am [Internet]. 1986 Dec [cited 2018 Apr 14];68(9):1348–53. Available from: http://www.ncbi.nlm.nih.gov/pubmed/3782206.

3. Shadgan B, Pereira G, Menon M, et al. Risk factors for acute compartment syndrome of the leg associated with tibial diaphyseal fractures in adults. J Orthop Traumatol [Internet]. 2015 Sep 28 [cited 2018 Apr 14];16(3):185–92. Available from: http://www.ncbi.nlm.nih.gov/pubmed/25543232.

4. DeLee JC, Stiehl JB. Open tibia fracture with compartment syndrome. Clin Orthop Relat Res [Internet]. 1981 Oct [cited 2018 Apr 8];(160):175–84. Available from: http://www.ncbi.nlm.nih.gov/pubmed/7026116.

5. Hope MJ, McQueen MM. Acute compartment syndrome in the absence of fracture. J Orthop Trauma [Internet]. 2004 Apr [cited 2018 Apr 8];18(4):220–4. Available from: http://www.ncbi.nlm.nih.gov/pubmed/15087965.

6. von Keudell AG, Weaver MJ, Appleton PT, et al. Diagnosis and treatment of acute extremity compartment syndrome. Lancet [Internet]. 2015 Sep 26 [cited 2018 Apr 8];386(10000):1299–310. Available from: http://www.ncbi.nlm.nih.gov/pubmed/26460664.

7. Schmidt AH. Acute compartment syndrome. Injury [Internet]. 2017 Jun [cited 2018 Apr 15];48:S22–5. Available from: http://www.ncbi.nlm.nih.gov/pubmed/28449851.

8. Mubarak SJ, Owen CA, Hargens AR, et al. Acute compartment syndromes: diagnosis and treatment with the aid of the wick catheter. J Bone Joint Surg Am [Internet]. 1978 Dec [cited 2018 Apr 8];60(8):1091–5. Available from: http://www.ncbi.nlm.nih.gov/pubmed/721856.

9. Ulmer T. The clinical diagnosis of compartment syndrome of the lower leg: are clinical findings predictive of the disorder? J Orthop Trauma [Internet]. 2002 Sep [cited 2018 Apr 8];16(8):572–7. Available from: http://www.ncbi.nlm.nih.gov/pubmed/12352566.

10. Shuler FD, Dietz MJ. Physicians' ability to manually detect isolated elevations in leg intracompartmental pressure. J Bone Joint Surg Am [Internet]. 2010 Feb [cited 2018 Apr 8];92(2):361–7. Available from: http://insights.ovid.com/crossref?an=00004623-201002000-00013.

11. Collinge C, Attum B, Tornetta P, et al. Acute compartment syndrome: an expert survey of Orthopedic Trauma Association (OTA) members. J Orthop Trauma [Internet]. 2018 Jan 24 [cited 2018 Apr 8];1. Available from: http://insights.ovid.com/crossref?an=00005131-900000000-98659.

12. McQueen MM, Duckworth AD, Aitken SA, et al. The estimated sensitivity and specificity of compartment pressure monitoring for acute compartment syndrome. J Bone Joint Surg [Internet]. 2013 Apr 17 [cited 2018 Apr 14];95(8):673–7. Available from: http://www.ncbi.nlm.nih.gov/pubmed/23595064.

13. McQueen MM, Court-Brown CM. Compartment monitoring in tibial fractures. The pressure threshold for decompression. J Bone Joint Surg Br [Internet]. 1996 Jan [cited 2018 Apr 15];78(1):99–104. Available from: http://www.ncbi.nlm.nih.gov/pubmed/8898137.

14. Whitney A, O'Toole RV, Hui E, et al. Do one-time intracompartmental pressure measurements have a high false-positive rate in diagnosing compartment syndrome? J Trauma Acute Care Surg [Internet]. 2014 Feb [cited 2018 Apr 14];76(2):479–83. Available from: https://insights.ovid.com/crossref?an=01586154-201402000-00033.

15. Harris IA, Kadir A, Donald G. Continuous compartment pressure monitoring for tibia fractures: does it influence outcome? J Trauma Inj Infect Crit Care [Internet]. 2006 Jun [cited 2018 Apr 14];60(6):1330–5. Available from: https://insights.ovid.com/crossref?an=00005373-200606000-00025.

16. Bistolfi A, Massazza G, Verné E, et al. Antibiotic-loaded cement in orthopedic surgery: a review. ISRN Orthop. [Internet]. 2011 Aug 7 [cited 2018 Mar 9];2011:1–8. Available from: https://www.hindawi.com/archive/2011/290851/.

17. Schaffzin JK, Prichard H, Bisig J, et al. A collaborative system to improve compartment syndrome recognition. Pediatrics [Internet]. 2013 Dec 1 [cited 2018 Apr 20];132(6):e1672–9. Available from: http://pediatrics.aappublications.org/cgi/doi/10.1542/peds.2013-1330.

18. Cascio BM, Pateder DB, Farber AJ, et al. Improvement in documentation of compartment syndrome with a chart insert. Orthopedics [Internet]. 2008 Apr [cited 2018 Apr 20];31(4):364. Available from: http://www.ncbi.nlm.nih.gov/pubmed/19292285.

19. Schmidt AH, Bosse MJ, Frey KP, et al. Predicting Acute Compartment Syndrome (PACS): the role of continuous monitoring. J Orthop Trauma [Internet]. 2017 Apr [cited 2018 Apr 15];31 Suppl 1:S40–7. Available from: http://insights.ovid.com/crossref?an=00005131-201704001-00009.

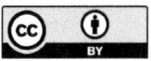

Chapter 17
Novel Modalities to Diagnose and Prevent Compartment Syndrome

Andrew H. Schmidt

Background

Acute compartment syndrome (ACS) of an extremity following trauma remains a diagnostic and therapeutic enigma. This phenomenon is because the clinical signs and symptoms of ACS are variable and nonspecific, and there are multiple causes of ACS after trauma (Table 17.1). Furthermore, the pathophysiology of ACS is poorly understood, which leads to confusion regarding the ideal diagnostic strategy. For decades now, ACS has been considered to be a pressure-related pathophysiologic

Table 17.1 Causes of acute compartment syndrome	Causes of acute compartment syndrome after trauma
	1. Accumulation of mass within the muscle compartment
	Bleeding
	Edema
	Tissue injury caused by direct trauma
	Inflammation and/or toxins
	Postischemic reperfusion
	Insertion of internal fixation hardware
	2. Reduction of compartment volume
	External compression from bandages, splints, casts
	Changes in the limb length related to fracture treatment
	External fixation
	Traction
	Internal fixation

A. H. Schmidt (✉)
University of Minnesota, Minneapolis, MN, USA

Department of Orthopedic Surgery, Hennepin Healthcare, Minneapolis, MN, USA
e-mail: schmi115@umn.edu

© The Author(s) 2019
C. Mauffrey et al. (eds.), *Compartment Syndrome*,
https://doi.org/10.1007/978-3-030-22331-1_17

169

process, with diagnostic recommendations largely based on pressure thresholds – either the absolute intracompartment pressure (ICP) or some measure of the perfusion pressure (defined as the difference between ICP and the patient's blood pressure). However, defining a single pressure threshold that accurately defines when fasciotomy is needed has not proven possible, and multiple studies suggest that clinical use of such thresholds leads to overtreatment [1–3].

Current treatment of ACS is surgical fasciotomy, which if not performed before the onset of cellular necrosis results in intractable pain, muscle fibrosis and contracture, and sensory deficits. Fasciotomy restores perfusion by increasing compartment volume so that the ICP falls, allowing tissue perfusion to be restored in viable vascular beds. This benefit is consistent with the traditional view of ACS as a "pressure problem." However, it is more appropriate to consider ACS as a metabolic problem, and both diagnostic and therapeutic strategies aimed at assessing cellular viability and reversing metabolic abnormalities may not only make our diagnosis of ACS more precise but also provide opportunities for less invasive ways to prevent ACS and mitigate the sequelae of ACS when it does occur.

New Concepts in ACS Pathophysiology

Compartment syndrome has been considered to be the result of tissue ischemia caused by decreased perfusion of the limb from elevated ICP, which may occur from any one of the several mechanisms: arterial spasm, collapse of arterioles, or collapse of the venous system. However, a recent series of publications by researchers in London, Ontario, Canada, has shown that ACS is accompanied by both a local and a systemic inflammatory response that may play a significant role in the pathogenesis of ACS and the resultant tissue damage [4–9]. This knowledge "opens the door" to using inflammatory mediators as potential biomarkers for understanding the progression or resolution of ACS and anti-inflammatory therapies as either primary or adjunctive medical therapy for ACS.

In a series of animal studies [4–9], the relationship between elevated ICP and the inflammatory response on skeletal muscle microcirculation and cell viability was measured in rats using intravital videomicroscopy. In one study, the level of tissue injury in an experimental compartment syndrome was compared between normal rats and those with neutropenia induced by injection of high-dose cyclophosphamide [5]. Muscle cellular injury was reduced more than 50% in neutropenic compared to healthy rats. Furthermore, the control rats had higher tissue injury ($23.0\% \pm 4.0\%$ of cells) compared to the neutropenic group ($7.0\% \pm 1.0\%$ of cells) after 90 minutes of elevated ICP ($p = 0.00005$) [5].

In a second study using a similar experimental model, local and systemic cytokine activation was measured and showed that animals with ACS have a systemic inflammatory response in addition to the local injury [4]. Remote organ damage was measured in the liver using intravital videomicroscopy techniques. Leukocyte activation, increased serum TNF-α levels, and necrotic hepatocytes were noted after 2 hours of ACS, all indicating systemic effects from ACS induced in one limb.

These same researchers have also demonstrated that attenuation of the inflammatory response may be beneficial in cases of ACS. Manjoo et al. [9] studied the effect of indomethacin on the level of tissue injury measured in rats with induced elevations in ICP for 45 or 90 minutes. Tissue injury was reduced almost to baseline levels in rats that were pretreated with indomethacin; a smaller benefit was noted when indomethacin administration was delayed [9]. In another study using the same model, treatment with a different anti-inflammatory molecule (CO-releasing molecule 3) led to statistically significant improvement in the number of continuously perfused capillaries, resulted in decreased tissue injury, reversed the ACS-associated increase in TNF- α, and reduced leukocyte adherence [6].

This series of papers indicate that ACS is accompanied by a substantial inflammatory response in the involved limb that also affects other organ systems. This information suggests that mitigation of the tissue injury caused by ACS may be possible by decreasing inflammation. Further work to determine the benefits of inflammatory modulation in a larger animal model is necessary, followed by clinical research in humans. The ideal therapeutic agent, mode of delivery, and timing are all unknown questions at this time.

New Diagnostic Modalities

The traditional diagnosis of ACS has been based on the clinical examination, supplemented when needed by intracompartment pressure measurement. Newer diagnostic approaches to ACS include near-infrared spectroscopy (NIRS), biomarker analysis, and radiofrequency identification (RFID) implants. These new approaches are discussed in the following paragraphs.

NIRS

In the context of measuring tissue perfusion in possible cases of ACS, NIRS uses differential light reflection and absorption to estimate the proportion of hemoglobin saturated with oxygen approximately 2–3 cm below the surface of the skin [10–14]. The depth of tissue interrogation is determined by the distance between the light source and the receptor.

The potential use of NIRS to diagnose ACS is supported by preclinical studies. In 1999, Garr et al. induced compartment syndrome in anesthetized pigs and showed that NIRS was a better predictor of neuromuscular dysfunction than compartment perfusion pressure [10]. However, its clinical use has shown mixed success. A case report published in 2011 outlined the benefits of using NIRS in three cases of lower extremity ACS [13]. NIRS differentiated between adequately perfused lateral compartments and poorly perfused deep posterior compartments of one patient with ACS. In another unresponsive patient diagnosed with ACS on clinical means, NIRS was able to detect perfusion deficits. In a third patient, NIRS demonstrated changes in muscle perfusion due to anesthetic induction within seconds [13]. However, also in 2011, Bariteau et al. described seven patients with a clinical diagnosis of ACS who had oxyhemoglobin saturation (rSO_2) and ICP values measured in each compartment of the affected lower extremity before undergoing fasciotomy. No statistically significant association was observed between rSO_2 and ICP or perfusion pressure [11].

Many questions remain about the clinical use of NIRS in traumatized limbs for diagnosing ACS, such as the ideal penetration depth, the effect of skin pigmentation and subcutaneous fat, the effect of skin abrasion or degloving, and subcutaneous or intramuscular bleeding. It has been demonstrated that injured limbs have a hyperemic response to injury, resulting in increased rSO_2 values [14].

One large theoretic advantage of NIRS is its potential ability to demonstrate changes in tissue perfusion corresponding with the onset of ACS. However, continuous NIRS has not been as well studied. Two recent papers have reported on continuous NIRS in a clinical setting. Shuler et al. [15] reported on 109 patients who had NIRS recording of the tissue perfusion in all four leg compartments of both legs (anterior, lateral, superficial posterior, and deep posterior): 86 had unilateral leg injuries while 23 did not. Mean NIRS values were between 72% and 78% in injured legs, between 69% and 72% in uninjured legs, and between 71% and 73% in bilaterally uninjured legs. NIRS values were typically >3% higher in injured limbs without ACS than in uninjured compartments. In contrast, all seven limbs with clinically diagnosed ACS had at least one compartment where NIRS values were 3% or more below an uninjured control compartment [15].

One problem with NIRS that may be even more of an issue when using NIRS in a continuous manner is the reliability of data capture. Shuler et al. noted that "Missing data were encountered in many instances" [15]. Schmidt et al. [16] used blinded continuous NIRS and blinded continuous ICP monitoring in 191 patients with leg injuries [16]. Data capture was unreliable with NIRS, with simultaneous data available from both injured and control limbs just 9% of the expected time, comparted to 88% of the expected time with continuous ICP [16]. At this time, it is not clear whether these data-capture issues with NIRS represent clinically immature technology that needs further development for this purpose or represent fundamental problems using NIRS to measure soft tissue oxygenation when that same tissue has had traumatic injury [16].

Biomarkers

Markers of muscle injury or metabolic disturbances such as acidosis may be measured systemically or locally.

Odland et al. have applied tissue ultrafiltration (TUF) catheters to the problem of diagnosing and treating acute compartment syndrome [17, 18]. TUF uses small diameter, flexible, hollow fiber catheters connected to suction in order to remove interstitial fluid, which may contain biomarkers of injury and contribute volume to the muscle compartment. The possible therapeutic benefits of TUF are discussed later in this chapter. In their study, serum and ultrafiltrate levels of creatine kinase and lactate dehydrogenase were measured hourly. The study demonstrated that bio-marker concentrations were up to 80-fold higher in ultrafiltrate than in serum.

A promising metabolic marker for ACS is tissue pH, as measured by intracom-partment probes. Basic science studies done at the University of Aberdeen in Scotland have revealed a correlation between local pH and depletion of high-energy phosphate stores [personal communication, Alan Johnstone 2018]. These same researchers have demonstrated that in a small study continuous pH measurement may be better than continuous pressure measurement at diagnosing ACS [19]. Further research is ongo-ing that should better define the role of pH monitoring on this setting.

RFID Chips in Diagnosing Compartment Syndrome

Current methods of diagnosing ACS rely on catheters or sensors that must remain attached to the patient and are therefore subject to inadvertent removal or may inter-fere with aspects of patient care, such as transportation, imaging, splinting, or the performance of surgical procedures. An "always-on" device that can be applied in a minimally or noninvasive manner and that does not interfere with transportation or other care of the patient would be a significant advance. New sensor technology that utilizes radiofrequency electromagnetic fields (radiofrequency ID tags or RFIDs) to transfer data exists and is beginning to be used for monitoring physiological sys-tems [20]. Such devices do require a battery and are powered externally by the very fields used to read their data. RFID pressure sensors have been developed and used for compartment monitoring [20].

Potential Therapeutic Advances in Treating ACS

In at-risk or early phases of compartment syndrome, before tissue necrosis has started to occur, other means of improving tissue perfusion and oxygenation may exist. One method would be to increase the tolerance of the muscle to ischemia. Other areas of theoretical interest include methods to decrease intramuscular pres-sure (tissue ultrafiltration, foot pumps, mannitol, and diuretics), improving tissue oxygenation, mitigating the effects of ischemia (free-radical scavengers and other pharmacologic measures), and small-volume resuscitation with hypertonic saline.

Tissue Ultrafiltration

Compartment syndrome is associated with accumulation of mass within a muscle compartment of relatively fixed volume, which is what results in the progressive increase in intramuscular pressure, which eventually sets in motion the vascular embarrassment and associated metabolic changes that result in tissue death. By removing even small amounts of fluid, loss of the associated fluid mass within the compartment may decrease compartment pressures. In an animal study, the potential benefits of tissue ultrafiltration (TUF) were demonstrated [18]. A bilateral infusion model of compartment syndrome in the pig hindlimb was used; each animal had one control limb and one treatment limb. Muscle pressure was measured with an indwelling catheter. Three TUF catheters were inserted into the anterior compartment of each limb. The catheters in the treatment limb were connected to negative pressure suction. The ICP pressure was lower in the treated limbs, and the muscle histology was more normal in the treated limbs compared to the control legs [18]. This study was followed up with clinical research on TUF in a small human trial. A pilot study demonstrated the feasibility of TUF in ten patients with tibial shaft fractures treated with nailing [17]. A small-randomized clinical trial of TUF versus pressure monitoring alone was also performed [21]. Fourteen patients were randomized to two groups: one used TUF plus monitoring while the other was monitored alone. Anterior and deep posterior pressures were measured for 24 hours in all patients. Outcome measures between the two catheters were compared using T-tests. The mean intramuscular pressure was smaller than in the control group in both the anterior and posterior compartments. Because of insufficient power, these differences were not statistically significant. Interestingly, two patients in the control catheter group developed compartment syndrome – 8 and 16 hours after the initial surgery and catheter insertion. No compartment syndromes were diagnosed in the treatment group.

Hypothermia

Tissue cooling has been used to improve tissue viability in transplant and replant surgery and is of known value in treating soft tissue injury. Sanders and colleagues, using a well-developed rat model (as described in the "New Concepts in ACS Pathophysiology" section of this chapter), showed that hypothermia to 25 °C reduced tissue damage score by 50% and also seemed to attenuate the inflammatory response [22]. Although this information is interesting, at this time the role of induced hypothermia for treating ACS in humans is not defined.

Conclusion

New concepts and ideas about the pathophysiology of ACS show promise at developing more physiologic, targeted treatments. These developments include modulation of the inflammatory response and new diagnostic modalities. Moreover, these advancements all address the current shortcomings in the diagnostic armamentarium that trauma surgeons can use, and which should lead to more precise methods to diagnose ACS and less invasive ways to prevent and treat it. Many of the approaches discussed in this chapter may be used simultaneously, and a multimodality approach to diagnosis and therapy, for example, using tissue ultrafiltration, intermittent plantar compression, small-volume resuscitation, and pharmacologic therapy, may someday be able to supplant fasciotomy for many patients.

References

1. Janzing HMJ, Broos PLO. Routine monitoring of compartment pressure in patients with tibial fractures: beware of overtreatment! Injury. 2001;32:415–21.
2. Prayson MJ, Chen JL, Hampers D, et al. Baseline compartment pressure measurements in isolated lower extremity fractures without clinical compartment syndrome. J Trauma. 2006;60:1037–40.
3. Whitney A, O'Toole RV, Hui E, et al. Do one-time intracompartmental pressure measurements have a high false-positive rate in diagnosing compartment syndrome? J Trauma Acute Care Surg. 2014;76:479–83.
4. Lawendy A-R, Bihari A, Sanders DW, et al. Compartment syndrome causes systemic inflammation in a rat. Bone Joint J. 2016;98-B:1132–7.
5. Lawendy A-R, Bihari A, Sanders DW, et al. Contribution of inflammation to cellular injury in compartment syndrome in an experimental rodent model. Bone Joint J. 2015;97-B:539–43.
6. Lawendy AR, Bihari A, Sanders DW, et al. The severity of microvascular dysfunction due to compartment syndrome is diminished by the systemic application of CO-releasing molecules (CORM-3). J Orthop Trauma. 2014;28:e263–8.
7. Lawendy A-R, McGarr G, Phillips J, et al. Compartment syndrome causes a systemic inflammatory response and remote organ injury. J Bone Joint Surg Br. 2011;93-B(Suppl III):280.
8. Lawendy AR, Sanders DW, Bihari A, et al. Compartment syndrome-induced microvascular dysfunction: an experimental rodent model. Can J Surg. 2011;54:194–200.
9. Manjoo A, Sanders D, Lawendy A, et al. Indomethacin reduces cell damage: shedding new light on compartment syndrome. J Orthop Trauma. 2010;24:526–9.
10. Garr JL, Gentilello LM, Cole PA, et al. Monitoring for compartmental syndrome using near-infrared spectroscopy: a noninvasive, continuous, transcutaneous monitoring technique. J Trauma. 1999;46:613–6.
11. Bariteau JT, Beutel BG, Kamal R, et al. The use of near-infrared spectrometry for the diagnosis of lower-extremity compartment syndrome. Orthopedics. 2011;34:178.
12. Shuler MS, Reisman WM, Kinsey TL, et al. Correlation between muscle oxygenation and compartment pressures in acute compartment syndrome of the leg. J Bone Joint Surg Am. 2010;2:863–70.
13. Shuler MS, Reisman WM, Cole AL, et al. Near-infrared spectroscopy in acute compartment syndrome: case report. Injury. 2011;42:1506–8.
14. Shuler MS, Reisman WM, Whitesides TE, et al. Near-infrared spectroscopy in lower extremity trauma. J Bone Joint Surg Am. 2009;91-A:1360–8.
15. Shuler MS, Roskosky M, Kinsey T, et al. Continual near-infrared spectroscopy monitoring in the injured lower limb and acute compartment syndrome. An FDA-IDE trial. Bone Joint J. 2018;100-B:787–97.
16. Schmidt AH, Bosse MJ, Obremskey WT, et al. Continuous near-infrared spectroscopy demonstrates limitations in monitoring the development of acute compartment syndrome in patients with leg injuries. J Bone Joint Surg Am. 2018;100:1645–52.
17. Odland RM, Schmidt AH. Compartment syndrome ultrafiltration catheters: report of a clinical pilot study of a novel method for managing patients at risk of compartment syndrome. J Orthop Trauma. 2011;25:358–65.

18. Odland R, Schmidt AH, Hunter B, et al. Use of tissue ultrafiltration for treatment of compart-ment syndrome: a pilot study using porcine hindlimbs. J Orthop Trauma. 2005;19:267–75.
19. Elliott K (2014) Intramuscular pH: Diagnosing acute compartment syndrome with confi-dence," in Proceedings of the 2014 London EFORT Conference Trauma Session.
20. Harvey EJ, Sanders DW, Shuler MS, et al. What's new in acute compartment syndrome? J Orthop Trauma. 2012;26:699–702.
21. Agudelo JF, Morgan SJ, Schmidt AH, et al. Management of acute compartment syndrome: randomized clinical trial evaluating a novel compartment syndrome catheter. OTA Annual Meeting, Ottawa, CAN, Oct. 2005.
22. Sanders DW, Chan G, Badhwar A. Hypothermia in compartment syndrome. J Bone Joint Surg Br. 2011;93-B(SUPP III):280.

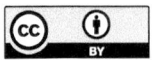

Corrections to: Fasciotomy Wound Management

Vasilios G. Igoumenou, Zinon T. Kokkalis, and Andreas F. Mavrogenis

Correction to:
C. Mauffrey et al. (eds.), *Compartment Syndrome*,
https://doi.org/10.1007/978-3-030-22331-1_9

One of the author's family name had been missed out in the References section (#1) in Chapter 9. This has now been corrected.

McLaughlin N, Heard H, Kelham S. Acute and chronic compartment syndromes: know when to act fast. JAAPA. 2014;27(6):23–6. https://doi.org/10.1097/01. JAA.0000446999.10176.13.

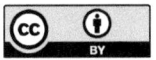
The updated online version of this chapter can be found at
https://doi.org/10.1007/978-3-030-22331-1_9

Index

© The Editor(s) (if applicable) and The Author(s) 2019
C. Mauffrey et al. (eds.), *Compartment Syndrome*,
https://doi.org/10.1007/978-3-030-22331-1